COGNITIVE THERAPY
FOR CHALLENGING PROBLEMS

©2005 Judith S. Beck
Published by The Guilford Press
A Division of Guilford Publications, Inc.
72 Spring Street, New York, NY 10012
www.guilford.com

Paperback edition 2011

Printed in the United States of America

This book is printed on acid-free paper.

Last digit is print number: 9 8 7 6 5

Library of Congress Cataloging-in-Publication Data
Beck, Judith S.
  Cognitive therapy for challenging problems: what to do when the basics don't work / Judith S. Beck; foreword by Aaron T. Beck.
    p. cm.
  Includes bibliographical references and index.
  ISBN 978-1-59385-195-8 (cloth: alk. paper)
  ISBN 978-1-60918-990-7 (paperback: alk. paper)
  1. Cognitive therapy. 2. Psychotherapist and patient. I. Title.
  RC489.C63B433 2005
  616.89′142–dc22
                                                    2005007221

To my family

About the Author

Judith S. Beck, PhD, is President of the Beck Institute for Cognitive Therapy (*www.beckinstitute.org*) and Clinical Associate Professor of Psychology in Psychiatry at the University of Pennsylvania School of Medicine. She has written nearly 100 articles and chapters as well as several books for professionals and consumers; has made hundreds of presentations, nationally and internationally, on topics related to CBT; and is the codeveloper of the Beck Youth Inventories and the Personality Belief Questionnaire. Dr. Beck is a founding fellow and past president of the Academy of Cognitive Therapy.

Foreword

This volume by Dr. Judith S. Beck is a major contribution to the literature addressing cognitive therapy with patients who have difficult problems. Through her own work with patients and her supervision of other therapists, Dr. Beck has been able to delineate the typical problems that thwart the progress of therapy and discourage therapist and patient alike. Until fairly recently these problems were considered manifestations of "resistance," "negative transference reactions," or "passive–aggressive tendencies" by many therapists. In response, many therapists are inclined to simply throw up their hands in frustration, not knowing what to do next.

Instead of yielding to these obstacles in therapy, Dr. Beck has consistently reframed these difficulties as identifiable, well-recognized problems with specific boundaries and characteristics. By categorizing the problems into specific domains, she has provided a readily available key to their complexities. Dr. Beck has thus drawn on her vast experience to outline the appropriate approach for each of the difficulties: (1) conceptualizing the problem in terms of the patient's developmental history, core beliefs and assumptions, and dysfunctional cognitions and behaviors, and (2) designing relevant strategies and techniques to solve the problem. Since each problem is different, it is necessary for therapists to adapt their therapeutic strategies accordingly, as artfully outlined in this volume.

The burden on the therapist was not always as heavy. In the early years of cognitive therapy, we were able to focus simply on our patients' here-and-now problems and prescribe relevant techniques. For depressed patients, this consisted of behavioral activation through activity scheduling, completing dysfunctional thought records, and engaging in practical problem solving. In general, the depression (or anxiety disorder) had disappeared by the 10th session and we scheduled one more simply for relapse prevention (Rush, Beck, Kovacs, & Hollon, 1977). As time passed, however, the duration of sessions for patients with comorbid disorders or complex or chronic problems (such as those described in this book) extended to 15, 20, 25, or even more sessions.

The patients began to receive the diagnosis of personality disorder in addition to their depression, anxiety, or panic disorder. Today the average patient seeking treatment at the Beck Institute for Cognitive Therapy is receiving at least two psychotropic medications and presents a history of limited response to pharmacotherapy or previous psychotherapy. At the core of this relative impermeability to therapy is the diverse array of therapy problems so beautifully described by Dr. Beck.

Where have all the "easy cases" gone? We have puzzled over this mystery for some time. Our hunch is that most patients respond reasonably well to their first-line treatment—by primary care doctors or psychopharmacologists. The relative nonresponders eventually may be referred for cognitive therapy, which now represents a secondary—or even a tertiary—level of care. As reconceptualized by Dr. Beck, the problems of the patients in this group represent a challenge rather than a burden to the psychotherapist. She has succeeded admirably in showing the therapist how to meet this challenge as well as to relieve the burden.

Of course, I cannot complete this introduction without acknowledging my special relationship to Dr. Judith Beck. As is generally known, she was practically born into cognitive therapy. By the time she reached adolescence, my theory and practice of cognitive therapy had pretty much crystallized but there was practically nobody with whom I could check out my ideas. So I tried them out on my teenage daughter, who reassured me, "They make good sense, Dad." I made no efforts to encourage her to follow in my footsteps. After college she embarked on a successful career in special education. However, I imagine that cognitive therapy still "made good sense" since she decided to make a career shift into clinical psychology with a specialty in cognitive therapy. I am particularly proud of her first volume, *Cognitive Therapy: Basics and Beyond*, designed primarily for beginning cognitive therapists, and the present volume for advanced cognitive therapists. Both volumes will, I am certain, be a boon for therapists and patients alike.

AARON T. BECK, MD

REFERENCE

Rush, A. J., Beck, A. T., Kovacs, M., & Hollon, S. (1977). Comparative efficacy of cognitive therapy and imipramine in the treatment of depressed outpatients. *Cognitive Therapy and Research, 1,* 17–37.

Acknowledgments

How lucky I am to have Aaron Beck as my father, mentor, and teacher. Obviously I would not have written this book without his development of the field of cognitive therapy. Reading his collected works; discussing research, theory, and practice with him; observing him treating patients; watching him teach; and reviewing cases with him have helped shape my development as a cognitive therapy practitioner and teacher. I, like countless mental health professionals and clients, owe him an enormous debt of gratitude.

Many other individuals have also played an important role in the writing of this book. First there are my primary coaches, cheerleaders, and feedback providers: my mother, Phyllis Beck; my friend, colleague, and right-hand woman, Naomi Dank; my husband, Richard Busis. I'd also like to acknowledge my children, Sarah, Debbie, and Sam, who managed to grow up in the many years it took me to write this book; they don't know how much I've learned from them.

I also owe thanks to my colleagues Andrew Butler, Norman Cotterell, Leslie Sokol, and Chris Reilly at the Beck Institute. Discussing cases with them over the past 10 years has helped me sharpen my thinking and expand my horizons. My colleague Cory Newman made many valuable suggestions that enriched the manuscript, as did my extremely patient, kind, and very helpful editor and friend, Kitty Moore, of The Guilford Press. I am also grateful to my patients, supervisees, students, and the innumerable workshop participants who provided me with case examples of challenging problems.

Contents

CHAPTER 1

Identifying Problems in Treatment

As I was writing *Cognitive Therapy: Basics and Beyond*, I knew a "standard" cognitive therapy text could not cover the multiplicity of difficulties presented by many patients. Some patients just fail to progress when therapists use standard treatment. Some patients do not seem to grasp or are unable to implement standard therapeutic techniques. Some patients seem to be unwilling to engage sufficiently in treatment. Others seem to cling to their long-standing distorted beliefs about themselves, other people, and their worlds. Treatment must be varied for these patients. But how does a therapist know when and how to alter treatment?

When experienced cognitive therapists encounter a challenging therapeutic problem, they seem to understand intuitively what they need to do. After repeated requests for a book that deals with these kinds of problems, I began to more closely observe the moment-to-moment decisions I make during therapy sessions. What may appear to be an intuitive process of decision making is actually based on a continuous ongoing conceptualization of patients, their diagnosis, and their experience of the therapy session. In addition to observing my own work, I have also been very fortunate to be able to observe and closely analyze therapy sessions conducted by my father, Aaron T. Beck, MD, as well as those conducted by my colleagues and supervisees.

This book reflects what I have learned since the publication of *Cognitive Therapy: Basics and Beyond*. That book presents step-by-step methods for using cognitive therapy with patients who exhibit straightforward cases of depression and anxiety and is an important precursor to this book, which is designed to help therapists figure out what to do when the basics do not seem to work.

Many complex reasons account for the difficulties patients present in treatment. Some problems are outside a therapist's control—for example, a patient may not be able to come to treatment frequently enough due to financial constraints, or a patient's environment may be so deleterious that psychotherapy is of limited utility to him or her. But most problems are within, or at least partially within, a therapist's control. Difficulties may arise because of patients' distorted beliefs (e.g., "If I get better, my life will get worse") and/or because of therapist error (e.g., using a standard treatment for depression with a patient who is actually suffering from another disorder).

At literally hundreds of workshops that I have conducted in the past decade, I have asked mental health professionals to describe the specific problems they have experienced with their patients. I have reached two important conclusions. First, many therapists initially tend to describe difficulties in global terms that do not clearly define the problem, asserting, for example, that a patient is "resistant." Second, when therapists do specify problems, they tend to mention the same kinds of difficulties time and again: patients who do not do homework, patients who become angry at the therapist, patients who engage in self-defeating behaviors between sessions, and so on. I have discovered that many therapists need to learn to state patients' difficulties in behavioral terms, to understand relevant difficulties within a cognitive framework, and to devise strategies based on their specific conceptualization of an individual patient. This book teaches the therapist to:

- Specify problems (and determine the degree of control a therapist has to ameliorate them).
- Conceptualize individual patients, including those with Axis II disorders.
- Deal with patients' problematic reactions to therapists and vice versa.
- Set goals, structure sessions, do problem solving, and enhance homework adherence (including behavior change) for patients with challenging problems.
- Identify and modify entrenched dysfunctional cognitions (automatic thoughts, images, assumptions, and core beliefs).

Appendix A outlines opportunities for continuing professional growth in cognitive therapy. Sometimes there is just no substitute for hands-on training and supervision.

SPECIFYING PROBLEMS

Even the most experienced cognitive therapists have difficulty with some patients. It may be tempting to blame our patients for presenting challenging problems and to attribute their attitudes and dysfunctional behaviors to their own character flaws. It is usually not helpful, though, to view the problem broadly, labeling patients as "resistant," "unmotivated," "lazy," "frustrating," "manipulative," or "stuck." Global descriptions such as "The patient doesn't seem to want to be in therapy" or "The patient expects me to do all the work" are also too general to be useful. It is far more productive to *specify the behaviors* that interfere with therapeutic progress and to adopt a problem-solving stance. Therapists can precisely define the difficulty by asking:

> ■ "What specifically does the patient say or do (or not say or do) within the therapy session—or between sessions—that is a problem?"

Typical problematic behaviors that some patients display *in* session include:

- Insisting they cannot change or that therapy cannot help them.
- Failing to set goals or contribute to the agenda.
- Complaining about, denying, or blaming others for their problems.
- Presenting too many problems or jumping from crisis to crisis.
- Refusing to answer questions or going off on tangents.
- Arriving late for or skipping sessions.
- Demanding entitlements.
- Becoming angry, upset, critical, or nonresponsive.
- Being unable or unwilling to change their cognitions.
- Being inattentive or continually interrupting the therapist.
- Lying or avoiding the disclosure of important information.

Many patients also display dysfunctional behavior *between* sessions, such as:

- Not doing homework.
- Failing to take needed medication.
- Abusing drugs or alcohol.
- Repeatedly calling the therapist while in crisis.
- Engaging in self-harming behaviors.
- Injuring others.

Suicide attempts require immediate crisis intervention and assessment at an emergency room (and are beyond the scope of this book).

CASE EXAMPLE

Andrea, a patient with bipolar disorder, posttraumatic stress disorder, and borderline personality disorder was recently released from hospital following a suicide attempt. She has just started treatment with a new outpatient therapist. From the beginning, Andrea distrusts her new therapist and is hypervigilant for harm. She is guarded, resists setting goals, and repeatedly states that therapy cannot help her. She often becomes upset with her therapist, attributing negative motives to her and blaming her for causing Andrea distress. She refuses to do homework assignments or to take the medication her psychiatrist has prescribed for her.

When trying to determine how best to treat patients who, like Andrea, present a host of challenging problems, it is important to assess whether difficulties in therapy are related to a number of different possibilities:

- Patient pathology
- Therapist error
- Factors *inherent* in treatment (including level of care, format of therapy, and frequency of sessions), and/or
- Factors *external* to treatment (including the presence of organic disease, the toxicity of the patient's environment, or the need for adjunctive treatments)

Many of the problems described in this book are related to the first factor: patient pathology. Patients who present a challenge in treatment often demonstrate long-standing difficulties in their relationships, in their work, and in managing their lives. They usually have very negative ideas about themselves, others, and their worlds—views that they developed in and have maintained since childhood or adolescence. When these beliefs dominate their perceptions, patients then tend to perceive, feel, and behave in highly dysfunctional ways, across time and across situations—including in the therapy session itself. It is important for therapists to recognize the activation of these beliefs and to determine when and how therapy should be adjusted in response to them. Patients may also present challenges because of the nature of their disorder—for example, due to the ego-syntonicity of anorexia or the biologically influenced mood swings of bipolar disorder. Specialized treatment is necessary for these patients, too.

Other problems arise, however, because of missteps in treatment, when therapists fail to implement standard therapy appropriately. And some problems are due to a combination of the two. Yet, before assuming that a difficulty stems primarily from the patient's pathology or from mistakes made by the therapist, it is essential to specify the problem, consider its frequency and breadth, and assess what other factors may be involved. The rest of this chapter describes how to:

- Determine the extent of a problem or problems.
- Consider factors external to the therapy session.
- Diagnose therapist error.
- Identify patients' dysfunctional beliefs.
- Distinguish therapist error from patients' dysfunctional beliefs.

The final section describes what therapists can do to avoid therapeutic problems in the first place.

CONSIDERING THE EXTENT OF A PROBLEM

Therapists need to analyze problems that arise in treatment, assessing the severity and frequency of a problem before deciding what to do. They should ask themselves:

■ "Is this a problem that arises briefly within one session?"
■ "Is it a problem that persists within a session?"
■ "Or does the problem arise in many sessions?"

Mild problems may not need to be directly addressed, at least initially. George, a high school student, grimaced and rolled his eyes at the beginning of his first two therapy sessions. His therapist did not acknowledge George's behavior. Instead she took care to be appropriately empathic, with the goal of demonstrating to him that she was not going to be like other controlling adults in his life. She also helped him set goals that *he* wanted to reach, not necessarily those that others had laid out for him. By the middle of their second session, George was able to see that his therapist had much to offer him and his negative reactions ceased.

Some problems are fairly specific and isolated, and can be addressed through simple problem solving. Jerry became annoyed when his therapist asked him to complete weekly symptom checklists. He and his therapist compromised by having him rate his mood on a 10-point scale instead. Holly needed help figuring out how she could obtain childcare for her young children so she could attend sessions regularly and on time.

Other problems are more prominent in a session and may require various solutions. When Toni's therapist tried to help her evaluate a rigid belief, the patient was unable to see the situation in a different light. Her therapist simply said, "It doesn't sound as if this [discussion] is helpful right now. How about if we move on to [the next problem on the agenda]?" Bob looked distressed when his therapist interrupted him for the third time. Having ascertained that his distress was indeed related to the interruptions, his therapist apologized and suggested that he speak uninterruptedly for the next 5–10 minutes. In both cases, the therapist's change of plan solved the problem.

Sometimes the problem is with the session as a whole. Lucy felt worse toward the end of the session than when she first walked in. The therapist correctly attributed her distress to the continued activation of her core belief of worthlessness. They agreed to spend the last few minutes of each session talking conversationally about one of Lucy's interests (movies) so that Lucy could leave the session feeling less distressed. Margaret seemed irritable for the first part of her therapy session. In response to her complaint that her therapist had seemed unsympathetic, her therapist asked Margaret if she would like to express herself more fully while she, the therapist, listened carefully and refrained from problem solving until near the end of the session. Again, these problems were quickly dealt with.

An ongoing problem that cuts across sessions usually requires more time to discuss and problem-solve so the patient will be willing to continue and progress in therapy. Dean was continually annoyed with his therapist because he believed that she was trying to control him or put him down. His therapist needed to spend more time empathizing with him, eliciting and helping him to respond to dysfunctional ideas about *her* and doing problem solving in relation to the therapeutic relationship so that he could then focus his attention more fully on working on his everyday problems outside of therapy.

Most therapeutic problems can be resolved through problem solving, modifying patients' cognitions, or changing therapist behavior. When problems persist, it is important to assess a variety of factors that might be interfering with treatment, as described below.

CONSIDERING FACTORS EXTERNAL TO THE THERAPY SESSION

While some ongoing problems are related to the process and content of therapy sessions, others are influenced by external factors. The areas noted below are included in a checklist in Figure 1.1.

- Is the patient receiving an appropriate dose of therapy?

  Should the patient be seen more often? Less often?
  Should the patient be at a higher or lower level of care (outpatient vs. partial hospitalization vs. hospitalization)?

- Is the medication appropriate?

  If the patient is not taking medication, should he/she be?
  If the patient is taking medication, is he/she fully compliant?
  Is the patient having significant side effects?

- Could there be an undiagnosed organic problem?

  Should the patient have a physical checkup with a primary care physician or specialist?

- Is the format of therapy appropriate?

  Should the patient be in individual therapy?
  Group therapy?
  Couple therapy?
  Family therapy?

- Does the patient need adjunctive treatment?

  Should the patient be referred to a psychopharmacologist?
  Pastoral counselor?
  Nutritionist?
  Vocational counselor?

- Is the patient's current living or work environment too deleterious for him/her to progress?

  Should the patient seek another place to live for a period of time?
  Should the patient try to make significant changes in his/her job?
  Look for another job?

FIGURE 1.1. Factors to consider external to the therapy session.

Dose, Level of Care, Format of Treatment, and Adjunctive Treatment

Sometimes patients fail to make sufficient progress because the *"dose"* of therapy is not appropriate. Claudia, a highly symptomatic patient, improved considerably more quickly when her therapist encouraged her to come to therapy on a weekly, instead of every other week, basis. Janice, a patient whose anxiety disorder had remitted significantly, needed to be treated on a less frequent basis so she could put the skills she had learned in therapy into practice on her own, without relying so heavily on her therapist.

Patients may be receiving treatment at an inappropriate *level of care*. Larry, an unemployed patient with rapid-cycling bipolar disorder and frequent suicidal ideation, periodically deteriorated when treated on an outpatient basis and needed occasional hospitalization or a partial hospitalization program. Carol needed inpatient rehab to address her substance dependence before she could benefit sufficiently from outpatient treatment.

The *format* of therapy may be inappropriate for some patients. Russell, a patient with depression and significant Axis II pathology, made faster progress when he agreed to move from individual therapy to group cognitive therapy. He perceived that the experience of others in the group had been similar to his; therefore they had a high degree of credibility for him and he was more amenable to testing his thoughts and changing his behavior. Elaine, who had mild depression and anxiety along with borderline traits, had received several sessions of individual therapy. She began to improve significantly once her boyfriend joined her for couple therapy. Lisa, an oppositional teenager, did not benefit much from individual therapy by itself, especially since she tended to blame others and to minimize her responsibility for problems. But when her therapist alternated individual sessions with family sessions, Lisa began to improve.

Sometimes therapists do not have the special expertise that patients need and *adjunctive treatment* might be indicated. Some patients benefit significantly from additional forms of treatment, such as pastoral, vocational, or nutritional counseling. Many patients are helped from support and education in groups such as Alcoholics Anonymous, one of its variations, or self-help groups.

Biological Interventions

Many patients, especially those who have been taking medication for a period of time, benefit from a *medication consult* that may result in an increase, decrease, or change of medication. Joe, a severely depressed patient, was having a great deal of difficulty sleeping. Medication eased his sleep problem, allowing him to progress much better in therapy. Shannon, a patient with panic disorder, was taking a high dose of benzodiazapenes, which reduced her anxiety symptoms. She was not able to learn fully that these symptoms were not dangerous until she had tapered her medication. Nancy was experiencing sedating side effects from her antipsychotic medication and was unable to focus sufficiently in session (and while trying to do homework outside of session) until her medication was changed.

Patients can also have *undiagnosed medical problems* that need to be addressed. If they have not had a recent medical checkup, the therapist should suggest one. Mark presented with anxiety, irritability, weight loss, emotional lability, and impaired concentration. Fortunately, his therapist pushed him to see his primary care doctor, who then determined through a blood test that Mark was not suffering from depression but instead had hyperthyroidism. Alexandra, too, seemed depressed. She had a significant loss of interest in nearly all her activities, felt physically and mentally slowed down, couldn't sleep, and had gained weight. Her physician diagnosed her with hypothyroidism and her symptoms abated once she was treated with appropriate medication.

Other patients may present with symptoms that look as if they stem from psychiatric disorders but are actually the result of endocrine disorders, brain tumors, traumatic brain injuries, seizure disorders, central nervous system infections, metabolic or vitamin deficiency disorders, degenerative dementias, cerebrovascular diseases, or other medical conditions (see Asaad, 1995, for in-depth information on this topic).

Environmental Changes

Sometimes patients' environments are so harmful that therapeutic intervention must be combined with a change in environment. Rebecca, a severely depressed teenager with an eating disorder, lived with her single mother and three siblings. The household was chaotic; her mother was alcoholic and emotionally abusive and her mother's boyfriend was physically abusive to Rebecca. Rebecca made little headway in solving her problems until her therapist facilitated her move out of the house and helped her establish residence with an aunt. Ken, a patient with rapid-cycling bipolar disorder, which was only partially controlled, struggled daily with a job that was beyond his capabilities when he was symptomatic. He became more and more anxious, depressed, and suicidal. It was not until he took a much less demanding job that he was able to progress in therapy.

When patients fail to improve or pose another challenge to the therapist, it is essential to determine whether external factors such as those outlined above are involved. Addressing such difficulties, as well as exploring the possibility of therapist error or patients' dysfunctional beliefs, may be critical for patients to improve.

THERAPIST ERROR VERSUS PATIENTS' DYSFUNCTIONAL BELIEFS

Many problems that arise in therapy or between therapy sessions are related to mistakes the therapist has made, to patients' dysfunctional cognitions, or to both.

Is the Problem Related to Therapist Error?

Even well-experienced therapists inadvertently make mistakes. Typical errors, described throughout this book, include:

- An erroneous diagnosis (e.g., misdiagnosing panic disorder as a simple phobia).
- An incorrect formulation or conceptualization of the case (e.g., failing to recognize that anxiety, not depression, is primary for a particular patient or incorrectly identifying a patient's core beliefs).
- A failure to use one's formulation of the case and conceptualization of the patient to guide therapy (e.g., focusing on problems or cognitions that are not central to the patient's recovery).
- A faulty treatment plan (e.g., using principles of generalized anxiety disorder treatment for a patient with obsessive–compulsive disorder).
- A rift in the therapeutic alliance (e.g., the therapist has not recognized that the patient is becoming overly frustrated in the therapy session).
- An inadequate list of behavioral goals (e.g., the patient's goals are too broad).
- Inappropriate structure or pacing (e.g., the therapist fails to interrupt the patient enough to address an important problem thoroughly).
- Inadequate focus on solving current problems (e.g., the therapist initially focuses on a depressed patient's childhood trauma instead of focusing on helping her become more functional in her daily life).
- Incorrect implementation of techniques (e.g., devising an exposure hierarchy in which the first few steps are too difficult).
- Inappropriate homework (e.g., the therapist suggests a homework assignment that the patient is unlikely to complete).
- A failure to maximize the patient's memory of the session (e.g., the therapist fails to record for the patient, in writing or on tape, the most important points of the session).

It is often difficult for therapists to identify their own mistakes. Listening to an audiotape of a therapy session, or having a colleague listen to it, sometimes reveals these kinds of therapist errors, especially if the listener uses the Cognitive Therapy Rating Scale (Young & Beck, 1980) to assess the tape. This scale, available at www.academyofct.org along with an accompanying manual, is used to measure therapist competency in 11 areas. Often review of an audiotape alone, while necessary, is by itself inadequate and the therapist also needs to thoroughly review the case with a colleague or supervisor.

Is the Problem Related to Patients' Dysfunctional Beliefs?

Identifying the beliefs that may underlie patients' problems in therapy is described more fully in the next two chapters. Briefly, it is helpful to hypothesize patients' assumptions, then check out the hypotheses with the patient. To do so, the therapist might put him- or herself in the patient's shoes and ask two questions:

> ■ "If I [do this dysfunctional behavior], then what good thing happens?"
> ■ "If I [don't do this dysfunctional behavior], what bad thing might happen?"

Andrea, the patient described at the beginning of this chapter, often blamed others for her problems. Her assumptions were:

"If I blame others, I won't have to change. But if I acknowledge that I had a part in my difficulties, I'll feel bad, let others off the hook, and be responsible for changing—which I feel incapable of, anyway."

Andrea was quite guarded in what she said during the session because of the following assumptions:

"If I avoid answering [my therapist's] questions directly or get her off track, I'll be okay. But If I reveal myself to [my therapist], I'll feel exposed and vulnerable and she will judge me harshly and reject me."

A third set of assumptions accounted for Andrea's continual rationalizations to justify her lack of behavioral change. Underlying her failure to follow through with reasonable homework assignments were the following assumptions:

"If I maintain the status quo, I won't open myself up to greater pain. But if I try to make my life better, it will actually get worse."

Understanding the assumptions that patients hold often clarifies the reasons for their dysfunctional behavior. Testing and modifying these assumptions are often necessary before patients are willing to change.

Distinguishing between Problems Related to Therapist Error and Those Related to Patients' Dysfunctional Cognitions

The source of a problem is sometimes not readily apparent. Below are some typical difficulties that arise with patients who present challenging problems and examples of both therapist errors and patients' dysfunctional thoughts or beliefs.

- *The patient doesn't contribute to the agenda.*
  Therapist error: The therapist has not asked the patient (as part of a homework assignment) to think about which problems she most wants help in solving.
  Patient's cognition: "It is useless to discuss this because my problems are insoluble."

- *The patient becomes upset when the therapist interrupts.*
  Therapist error: The therapist is interrupting too much or too abruptly and the patient reasonably feels uncomfortable.
  Patient's cognition: "My therapist interrupts me because he wants to control me."

- *The patient vigorously negates the therapist's views.*
  Therapist error: The therapist has expressed his views too forcefully or too early in therapy or his views are erroneous.
  Patient's cognition: "If I adopt my therapist's viewpoint it means my therapist has won and I have lost."

- *The patient complains about problems instead of engaging with the therapist in solving problems.*
  Therapist error: The therapist has not sufficiently socialized the patient to the process of therapy or does not interrupt the patient to steer him toward problem solving.
  Patient's cognition: "I shouldn't have to change."

- *The patient is inattentive.*
  Therapist error: The therapist has not adjusted treatment for a patient who has attentional difficulties or for a patient who is experiencing high levels of distress that interfere with processing.
  Patient's cognition: "If I listen to my therapist, I'll get too upset."

AVOIDING PROBLEMS IN THERAPY

Therapists can minimize the occurrence of problems by ensuring that they continuously follow some of the central precepts of cognitive therapy (described more fully in J. Beck, 1995):

1. Accurately diagnose and formulate the case.
2. Conceptualize the patient in cognitive terms.
3. Use the cognitive formulation and the individual conceptualization to plan treatment within and across sessions.
4. Build a strong therapeutic alliance.
5. Set specific behavioral goals.
6. Employ basic strategies.
7. Use advanced strategies and techniques.
8. Assess the effectiveness of interventions and of therapy.

These elements are briefly described below and illustrated throughout the book.

Diagnosis and Formulation

Since the focus of cognitive therapy treatment for one disorder may be significantly different from that of another, it is essential to conduct a thorough clinical assessment of patients that yields an accurate diagnosis. For example, the treatment for posttraumatic stress disorder differs in some important ways from the treatment of generalized anxiety disorder.

It is also important to formulate the case correctly. The most important cognitions in the treatment of panic disorder, for example, are the patient's catastrophic misinterpretation of symptoms (Clark & Ehlers, 1993). In depression, negative thoughts about the self, the world, and the future are most important to target (Beck, 1976). In obsessive–compulsive disorder, it is important not to focus heavily on modifying the *content* of patients' obsessive thoughts or images, but instead to modify their *appraisal* of their obsessive cognitions (Frost & Stekettee, 2002; Clark, 2004; McGinn & Sanderson, 1999). If a therapist employs a generic approach for patients, without varying it according to an individual patient's disorder, the patient is unlikely to make sufficient progress. Additional information about treatment manuals can be found at www.beckinstitute.org.

Therapists also must be aware of key issues affecting patients and their treatment, for example, their age, developmental level, intellectual level, cultural milieu, spiritual beliefs, gender, sexual orientation, physical health, and stage of life. Mia, for example, was Asian. Her therapist unwittingly alienated her by questioning her extremely strong cultural belief about the need to obey one's parents. Janet's therapist did not understand the grief she felt when her youngest child left home, and instead of empathizing and supporting her, tried to modify her thinking, which left Janet believing she was defective for having a normal, human reaction. Keith's therapist failed to take into account his aging patient's difficulty with mobility and memory and suggested homework assignments that were doomed to failure.

At times it becomes apparent even at the evaluation or first therapy session that treatment will need to be varied. Understanding that Andrea, described above, had borderline personality disorder with strong paranoid features helped her therapist think about how therapy with Andrea might have to be different from therapy with a patient who was experiencing a first episode of depression and who had no significant Axis II pathology.

Diagnosis and formulation of the case needs to be ongoing. A comorbid diagnosis may not, for example, be obvious at the start of treatment. Eleanor, a patient with depression and panic disorder, made some progress in therapy but then became stuck. It was not until her therapist realized that she also had a significant case of social phobia, and began treating her for it, that Eleanor began to improve again. The same was true for Rodney, who initially minimized the extent of his drug use.

Cognitive Conceptualization

Therapists need to develop and continually refine a cognitive conceptualization of the individual patient. The conceptualization, described in Chapter 2, helps therapists (and patients) understand why the patient currently reacts to situations and problems in a particular way and to identify the central cognitions and behaviors that are important to target in therapy. Patients may have any number of problems and problematic behaviors, thousands of automatic thoughts, many dozens of dysfunctional beliefs. Therapists must quickly identify the specific cognitions and behaviors most needing—and most amenable to—change.

Planning Treatment Across and Within Sessions

An accurate diagnosis and formulation of the case enables the therapist to devise a general treatment approach for the patient across sessions. An accurate, continuously evolving cognitive conceptualization enables the therapist to focus on the patient's most central problems, dysfunctional cognitions, and behaviors in each session. Treatment planning within sessions is illustrated throughout this book.

Building the Therapeutic Alliance

To engage fully in treatment, most patients need to feel that their therapists are understanding, caring, and competent. Yet even when their therapists display these characteristics, some patients react negatively—for example, they may become suspicious of their therapist's motives. Sometimes therapists need to vary their style, becoming more or less empathic, structured, didactic, confrontive, self-disclosing, or humorous. An autonomous patient, for example, may prefer his therapist to be business-like and slightly removed, while a sociotropic patient may respond better if his therapist is warm and friendly (Leahy, 2001). The ability to pinpoint, conceptualize, and overcome difficulties in the therapeutic relationship is essential to helping patients progress—and may help them improve other relationships as well, as described in Chapters 4 and 5.

Setting Specific Behavioral Goals

It is important for therapists to guide patients to identify specific goals they would like to reach as a result of therapy. Many patients initially state that they would like to feel happier or less dysphoric. These long-term goals are too broad to easily work toward and achieve. Therapists often have to ask patients what they would be *doing differently* if they were happier; the behaviors they state then become the short-term goals toward which patients work at each session.

Employing Basic Strategies

It is important to have patients engage in fundamental therapy tasks: identifying and responding to their automatic thoughts, completing homework assignments, scheduling activities (this task is especially important for depressed patients), and exposing themselves to feared situations (this task is especially important for patients with anxiety disorders). Therapists whose patients are highly resistant to doing such tasks may drop their focus on these essential activities altogether, when instead they should negotiate with their patients about improving adherence or help their patients respond to associated dysfunctional cognitions.

Using Advanced Techniques

Therapists often need to use a wide variety of techniques with patients. These techniques are typically cognitive, behavioral, problem solving, supportive, or interpersonal. Some techniques are emotional in nature (e.g., teaching emotional regulation skills to highly reactive patients or heightening affect in avoidant patients). Some are biological (e.g., ruling out an organic cause of symptoms, helping patients cope with medication side effects or a chronic medical condition). Some are environmental (e.g., helping an abused patient find another living situation). Some are experiential (e.g., restructuring the meaning of early trauma through imagery). Some are psychodynamic-like (e.g., helping patients correct their distorted beliefs about the therapist).

Therapists often need to devise new techniques on the spot to deal with the activation of patients' emotionally charged beliefs or, conversely, their avoidance of emotionally charged material (Newman, 1991; Wells, 2000). Nonstandard techniques are sometimes essential, for example, to maintain a strong therapeutic alliance or to help patients gain an emotional or gut-level change in belief.

Assessing the Effectiveness of Interventions and of Therapy

To gauge progress and plan treatment across and within sessions, it is essential to conduct a mood check at the beginning of each session (J. Beck, 1995), preferably accompanied by self administered scales such as the Beck Depression Inventory (Beck, Ward, Mendelson, Mock, & Erbaugh, 1961) or Beck Youth Inventories (J. Beck, Beck, & Jolly, 2000). In addition, it is important to assess progress during the therapy session itself. Standard techniques should be employed, such as asking patients to summarize periodically during the session or checking on the degree of negative emotion patients feel *before* and *after* discussing a problem in therapy (as well as the degree to which they believe their dysfunctional cognitions).

Change in the therapy session itself, however, is insignificant if patients return to the same negative thinking and mood once the session is over and/or they fail to make necessary behavioral change between sessions. An important part of gauging how well therapy is going is determining what constitutes reasonable progress for a patient. For many of the patients described in this book, progress was quite slow, but fairly steady, with setbacks along the way.

SUMMARY

Part of the art of conducting cognitive therapy lies in identifying problems in treatment, assessing the severity of the problems, and then specifying the source of the problems. Difficulties may be related to factors external to treatment (e.g., a deleterious environment), factors inherent in the treatment (e.g., an insufficient level of care), therapist error (e.g., incorrect implementation of techniques), and/or the patient's pathology (e.g., deeply entrenched beliefs). Outside consultation is sometimes necessary to diagnose a problem adequately. Creative solutions to typical difficulties are presented throughout this book. The next chapter, which addresses cognitive conceptualization, lays the groundwork for understanding why problems related to patients' pathology arise.

CHAPTER 2

Conceptualizing Patients Who Present Challenges

Cognitive conceptualization is the cornerstone of cognitive therapy. A sound conceptualization allows the therapist to guide treatment effectively and efficiently. Patients may enter therapy with many problems and may experience hundreds of dysfunctional cognitions in the course of their day or week that lead to distress and dysfunctional behavior. How do cognitive therapists decide what to focus on in therapy? In general, they focus on problems (situations, behaviors, symptoms) that are current, upsetting, and likely to bring further distress in the coming week. They also focus on cognitions (thoughts and beliefs) that are related to important problems, that are clearly distorted or dysfunctional, that seem amenable to change, and that involve recurrent themes in the patient's thinking (J. Beck, 1995).

Accurately assessing patients with challenging problems is often more complex than assessing patients with more straightforward difficulties. They frequently present with many more problems and dysfunctional beliefs (J. Beck, 1998; Beck, Freeman, Davis, & Associates, 2004). This chapter presents a method to organize the multitude of data that these patients present so therapists can more easily determine how to plan treatment. First a simplified version of the cognitive model is outlined. Then core beliefs, the most fundamental understandings of the self, others, and the world, are described, along with behavioral strategies and assumptions. A diagram to aid therapists in cognitive conceptualization is presented. Finally an elaborated description of the cognitive model, along with complex sequences of patients' thoughts and reactions to current situations are provided.

THE COGNITIVE MODEL—SIMPLIFIED

In its simplest form, the cognitive model suggests that people's perceptions of situations influence how they react. Andrea bristles at her therapist in their first session, as illustrated in the diagram below.

Situation

Therapist asks Andrea what her goals for therapy are.

Automatic Thoughts

"Why is she asking me that? It's so superficial. Setting goals won't help. My problems
are too deep. She should know that. Didn't she read the evaluator's report?
She probably thinks I'm just like everyone else. I'm not going to let her get away
with treating me like this."

Reaction

Emotional: Anger
Physiological: Tension in face, arms, shoulders
Behavioral: Shrugs, avoids eye contact, says nothing

Andrea continually experiences these kinds of thoughts and reactions, perceiving that she is being treated badly in situation after situation:

> "What's the use [of returning a defective radio to the store]? They won't believe me."
> "If I go [to a support group the therapist suggests], people will look down on me."
> "The checkout clerk is deliberately making me wait."
> "[My therapist] is patronizing me."

These thoughts, termed "automatic thoughts," pop up spontaneously; Andrea is not consciously trying to think in this way. Why does she have such negative thoughts? Andrea has basic or core beliefs that she is vulnerable, bad, and helpless. She believes that people are critical, harsh, and superior to her. These ideas act like a filter or a lens by which she appraises situations. What contributes to her therapist's difficulty in treating Andrea is that her dysfunctional beliefs become highly activated not

only in everyday life but also during therapy sessions, as illustrated in the
diagram below.

Core beliefs

"I am vulnerable, bad, helpless."
"Other people are critical, harsh, and superior to me."

Situation

Therapist and Andrea discuss her difficulties organizing and paying her bills.

Situation is perceived through lens of core beliefs

Automatic thoughts

"[My therapist] is thinking how stupid I am."
"How dare she judge me!"
↓

Reaction

Emotional: Anger
Physiological: Clenches her fist
Behavioral: Tells therapist that she's not being helpful

Initially therapy was quite difficult for both Andrea and her therapist. Andrea's negative beliefs frequently became activated. For example,
her therapist tries to set an agenda and asks Andrea which problem she
would like to work on. Andrea thinks, "This is useless. I'm too far gone. I
can't be helped." She then feels hopeless, slumps in her chair, and says, "I
don't know." When her therapist asks how she might spend her time differently (i.e., more productively) this week, Andrea thinks, "What is she
talking about? I can't change," and tells her therapist in a slightly hostile
tone, "I can't even *imagine* being able to get any more done." When her
therapist tries to help her evaluate one of her automatic thoughts by asking, "Is there any evidence that perhaps you could gain at least a little
sense of mastery by [doing a household chore]?," Andrea flatly answers
"No" in a tone of voice that warns the therapist not to push her further.

The Cognitive Conceptualization Diagram (J. Beck, 1995) in Figure 2.1 depicts Andrea more fully, showing how the basic conceptual
elements—core beliefs, assumptions, and coping strategies (described
below)—are linked to one another and to Andrea's childhood experience
and her current experience. This diagram is explicated more fully on
pages 28–31.

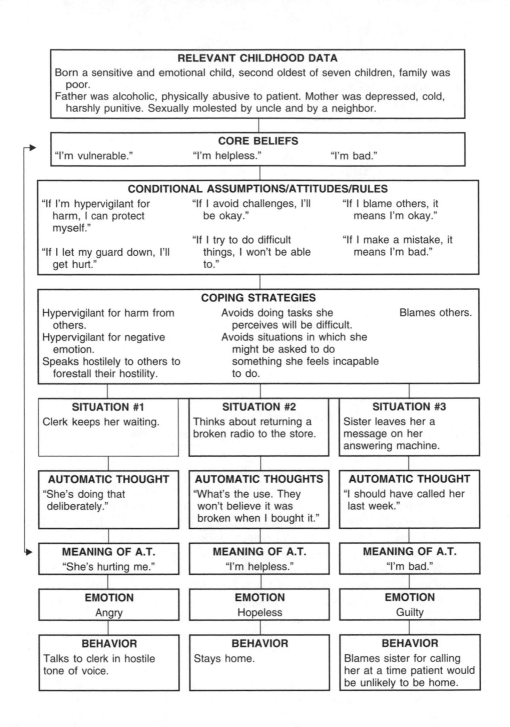

FIGURE 2.1. A Cognitive Conceptualization Diagram.

CORE BELIEFS

As children struggle to make sense of themselves, other people, and their worlds, they develop organizing concepts in their minds. They actively seek meaning and continually fit new data into existing schemas or templates. When childhood experience is perceived negatively, children often begin to attribute negative qualities to themselves. If they have enough meaningful positive experiences, they may see themselves in a negative light from time to time, but they basically believe that they are okay: reasonably effective, reasonably likable, reasonably worthwhile. If they do not, they may begin to develop negative views of themselves, their world, and/or other people.

If these negative concepts become organizing structures in their minds, children may begin to process information in a distorted and dysfunctional way, perceiving and focusing too strongly on the negative and discounting or failing to process positive information. Chapter 3 describes how this tendency becomes ingrained over time, leaving the child vulnerable to developing an Axis II disorder (Beck et al., 2004).

For example, Andrea's childhood was marked by a series of negative experiences, often occurring daily. Her family was impoverished. She had six brothers and sisters. Her father, an alcoholic, physically abused Andrea and her siblings. Her mother was chronically depressed, punitive, and emotionally and physically unaffectionate. Andrea was sexually molested at age 12 by an uncle and at age 13 by a neighbor. Not surprisingly, Andrea began to develop a number of negative ideas about herself, others, and her world. For example, she began to believe that she was helpless. Over time, this belief became structuralized in her mind.

Without conscious awareness, Andrea began to selectively focus on data that supported this idea, not only in interactions at home, but also in many situations and experiences outside of the house. She also began to distort information that did not fit with this belief. For example, when an older cousin praised her for helping take care of her siblings, Andrea thought he must have an ulterior motive for being nice to her. In addition, she simply did not recognize or put much weight on other positive data— for example, that she had some interactions with her peers and adults in which she was reasonably assertive and effective. Thus her belief that she was helpless became stronger, while a weak belief that she was effective became attenuated.

Core Beliefs about the Self

Individuals' negative beliefs about the self may be broadly conceptualized as falling into one of three categories: helplessness, unlovability, or worthlessness. For therapists to plan therapy effectively, they should start gathering data from their initial encounter with the patient and then generate hypotheses, based on the data and later confirmed by the patient, to determine whether the patient's beliefs involve a theme of helplessness, unlovability, worthlessness, or some combination of the three. Patients may have one major dysfunctional core belief or many; their core beliefs may fall primarily in one category described below or into more than one.

The *helpless* category has many different nuances but the major theme has to do with feeling ineffective in some way. Patients express this idea in different ways:

Helpless Core Beliefs

"I am inadequate, ineffective, incompetent; I can't cope."
"I am powerless, out of control; I can't change; I'm stuck, trapped, a victim."
"I am vulnerable, weak, needy, likely to be hurt."
"I am inferior, a failure, a loser, not good enough; I don't measure up to others."

Other patients, who believe they are *unlovable* or *unloved*, may or may not be overly concerned with being effective. They believe or fear that they will never obtain the intimacy and caring they want. They express this idea in the following ways:

Unlovable Core Beliefs

"I am unlikable, undesirable, ugly, boring; I have nothing to offer."
"I am unloved, unwanted, neglected."
"I will always be rejected, abandoned; I will always be alone."
"I am different, defective, not good enough to be loved."

Patients who see themselves as *worthless* may express the idea as:

Worthless Core Beliefs

"I am worthless, unacceptable, bad, crazy, broken, nothing, a waste."
"I am hurtful, dangerous, toxic, evil."
"I don't deserve to live."

The worthless beliefs often have a moral tone that differentiates them from the first two categories. When a patient expresses a belief of worthlessness, it is important to ascertain whether worthlessness is in and of itself the worst meaning to the patient, or whether unlovability or helplessness underlies the worthless belief. When Walter tells the therapist that he is worthless, his therapist probes further: "If it's true that you're worthless, what's the worst part of that? Is it that you can't be effective or productive—or that you'll never get the love you want?" Walter responded that the latter was worse. In contrast, when Sasha's therapist asked her what her core belief of worthlessness meant to her, she responded that neither was worse, that being worthless was in and of itself the worst possibility.

Why It Is Important to Identify the Category of a Patient's Beliefs

Rapid identification of the category in which a particular patient's beliefs falls helps guide treatment. In most cases, the therapist aims to elicit and modify patients' most central dysfunctional thoughts, beliefs, and behaviors. A patient who believes she is basically adequate and effective but whose belief of unlovability leads to significant distress should be encouraged to do behavioral experiments that involve taking steps toward connecting with others. Patients who believe that they are basically likable but are helpless or ineffective need to engage in a variety of mastery experiences.

Correctly conceptualizing the category or categories of patients' core beliefs is essential to conducting therapy effectively. One therapist, for example, miscategorized his patient's core belief. Edward had many automatic thoughts about losing his wife: "I'm such a bad husband. She [wife] is probably fed up. How much longer is she going to put up with me? She'll probably leave me." He also had thoughts about alienating others: "Chuck [the patient's best friend] must be tired of hearing me complain. He must think I'm really a loser. I'm sure he'd rather spend time with other people." Edward also had negative thoughts about his relationship with his mother: "I really should go and see her. She probably thinks I don't care about her."

The therapist believed that these thoughts indicated a strong belief of unlovability. He therefore focused on automatic thoughts about being a bad husband, friend, and son. He suggested homework assignments designed to help Edward connect more with loved ones and coworkers. Edward improved only slightly. Finally the therapist directly sought the *meaning* of Edward's thoughts: "If it were true that [your wife wants to leave you; your friend doesn't want to spend time with you; your mother thinks you don't care about her], what would be the worst part?" Edward answered, "I wouldn't be able to get along. I wouldn't have anyone to help me. I don't know what I'd do."

It became clear that Edward's overriding concern was *not* that he wouldn't have caring and intimacy (unlovability); rather, he was sure that if he alienated others and lost their support and help, he would not be able to cope (helplessness). Once his therapist oriented therapy toward evaluating automatic thoughts about being ineffective and inadequate and toward engaging in activities that gave him a sense of mastery, Edward's depression rapidly improved.

Why Patients Believe Their Core Beliefs So Strongly

Why do patients hold on to their beliefs so tenaciously, even in the face of extensive contradictory data? Robin believes, through and through, that she is bad, even though she has plenty of evidence to the contrary. She is a productive employee, her best friend treats her well and praises her frequently, she takes good care of her aged mother, she has a reasonable relationship with her sister, and her neighbors seem to like her. One strong contributing factor to her belief that she is bad is the way she processes information.

• *She continually selectively focuses on data that confirms her negative view.* She notices—and labels herself as bad—every time she perceives that she has made a mistake or has fallen short of her own (unrealistically high) expectations, every time she believes that she has fallen short of others' expectations for her, and every time she elicits a negative (or sometimes even a neutral) reaction from others. In the course of one day, for example, she labels herself as bad when she leaves her apartment without first straightening it up, when she arrives at work 10 minutes late (because her bus had been delayed), when her boss points out an error in her typing, and when she realizes she has forgotten to return a phone call to her mother.

• *She discounts data contrary to her belief.* When Robin notices positive data, she does not incorporate it in a straightforward way. When she goes to considerable effort to help her neighbor move some furniture, she thinks, "I really should have done more." When she helps her mother, she thinks, "I'm not doing this out of love, only out of obligation."

• *She fails to recognize contrary data.* Robin doesn't register the fact that she was on time for work 20 out of 21 days this month, that she was nice everyday to her coworkers, and that she frequently went out of her way to help her mother. Yet she would have concluded that she was bad had she *not* done these things.

This biased processing is not volitional. It occurs automatically, beyond Robin's awareness. Fortunately, Robin's therapist can help her understand her faulty information processing and counteract it (see Chapter 13). Robin learns to view her dysfunctional behavior and negative experiences less drastically. She also learns to respond adaptively to the discounting of her positive behavior and experiences and to identify and value positive data about herself that she had not previously recognized.

Core Beliefs about Others

Patients with challenging problems often perceive others in a rigid, overgeneralized, dichotomous way. They generally do not perceive that others are complex human beings who demonstrate traits to a greater or lesser degree in various situations. Rather, they categorize them, often in black-or-white terms. Frequently, their perceptions are exaggeratedly negative. People are demeaning, uncaring, hurtful, sinister, manipulative. Or they may see others in an unrealistically positive way, as superior, completely effective, lovable, worthwhile (while they themselves are not).

Core Beliefs about Their World

These patients often hold dysfunctional beliefs about their personal world. They may believe that they cannot get what they want from life because of the obstacles their world presents. They may phrase their beliefs as "The world is unfair, unfriendly, unpredictable, uncontrollable, dangerous." Usually these beliefs are quite global and overgeneralized.

Patients who hold a number of simultaneously activated core beliefs about themselves, others, and their worlds often believe that they have no safe haven in which to function. Andrea, for example, believes that her world is dangerous, that she is helpless, and that she is desperately in need of others to help her. Yet she simultaneously holds the belief that others are uncaring and hurtful. Thus, according to her gridlocked core beliefs, she must either be alone, helpless, and vulnerable or put herself at the mercy of malevolent others. Subjectively, she believes that she is doomed either way. Andrea finds others invalidating, which further confirms her web of dysfunctional beliefs.

BEHAVIORAL STRATEGIES

It is painful for people to hold extreme views of themselves, their worlds, and other people. Patients with challenging problems often develop certain patterns of behavior to protect themselves—to cope with or to compensate for their negative beliefs (Beck et al., 2004). Andrea, for example, believed that she was vulnerable and that other people were potentially hurtful. Therefore she developed a strategy of making herself hyperaware of others' behavior and keeping herself keenly alert for possible signs of malevolence. When she did perceive (or misperceive) mistreatment, her strategy was to verbally attack the other person.

Janice also believed that she was weak and that others were potentially hurtful. Her strategy, though, was to be hypervigilant for others' negative moods, to go overboard in pleasing and placating others, to subjugate her own desires, and to avoid conflict at all costs.

Patients with long-standing difficulties often develop these behavioral strategies as children or young adults. These patterns of behavior may (or may not) have been more functional for them earlier in life but generally become more and more maladaptive as the individual develops and enters new life situations. Overuse of their maladaptive strategies may protect them from an activation of their core belief at the moment. However, such behavior does not generally erode the core belief. When Andrea is verbally aggressive with others to avoid mistreatment, her core belief of vulnerability is not affected. She still believes, "If I hadn't [verbally attacked] them, they would have mistreated me. When Janice placated others, she still believed, "If I hadn't placated them, they would have hurt me."

Before therapy, patients vary in the degree to which they are aware of these patterns of behavior, but it is usually fairly easy to identify them. Understanding patients' core beliefs and assumptions is essential to discovering why patients behave in the way that they do. Their behavior makes sense given their beliefs.

Each personality disorder has its own set of central beliefs, assumptions, and strategies (described in Chapter 3). Examples of how different patients cope with the same core belief are provided below.

Core belief	Coping strategies
"I am inadequate."	Rely on others or try to overachieve.
"I am nothing."	Withdraw, avoid intimacy, be dramatic, or act entitled.
"I am vulnerable."	Act strong, dominate, or avoid any possibility of being hurt.

ASSUMPTIONS, RULES, AND ATTITUDES

One way of understanding patients' behavioral strategies is through examining a class of cognitions that fall between their more superficial automatic thoughts and their deeper core beliefs. Assumptions, rules, and attitudes comprise this intermediate group of beliefs (J. Beck, 1995; see also Chapter 12). *Conditional assumptions* demonstrate how one's behavioral strategies are connected to one's core beliefs. Patients generally believe that if they employ their coping strategies, they will be okay—but if they don't, their core beliefs will become evident or come true.

- "If I'm hypervigilant for harm and am hostile to people, I can protect myself, but if I'm not on guard, others will harm me."
- "If I keep the status quo, I'll be okay. But if I try to make changes, I won't be able to."
- "If I make a mistake, it means I'm bad."

One reason patients like Andrea are challenging to treat is that they often make the same assumptions about their therapist or about the process of therapy that they make about other people or other situations, and thus use their maladaptive coping strategies in treatment. At the beginning of therapy, Andrea was hypervigilant for harm and perceived that her therapist was trying to put her down, so she responded in a critical and hostile way. She believed that she was incapable of improving her life, so she resisted the therapist's attempts to try to get her to consider goals or to make small changes. Andrea also avoided revealing much about herself, believing that if she did, her therapist would reject her.

Patients also express the ideas contained in their assumptions in other forms, through *rules* and *attitudes*. The rule "I shouldn't reveal much about myself" might be associated with the assumption "If I reveal myself, I'll be rejected or hurt." The attitude "It's terrible to make a mistake" may be drawn from the assumption "If I make a mistake, it means I'm incompetent." It is often helpful to derive the assumption upon which a rule or attitude is based in order to test the idea more effectively.

Central Assumptions versus Subsets of Assumptions

Patients make thousands of assumptions. Thus it is critical to identify the broad, central ones so that the therapist can guide therapy effectively. The most important ones are usually tied to patients' core beliefs. It is also important to determine whether a new assumption that is uncovered in therapy represents a new theme that may need attention or whether the assumption is merely a subset of a previously identified central assumption.

For example, Alison held the following broad, central assumption:

"If I experience negative emotion, I'll fall apart."

Narrower subsets of this assumption were:

"If I focus on what my therapist is saying, I'll feel terrible and I won't be able to stand it."

"If I do my therapy homework, I'll have to think about my problems and I won't be able to tolerate the bad feelings that I'll have."

"If I think about [even gently] confronting my mother, I'll get so anxious I might go crazy."

In a later therapy session, as they were discussing how Alison might spend her weekend, she expressed another assumption:

"If I don't do what my sister wants, she'll feel bad."

The therapist had not previously recognized the theme inherent in this assumption. She wondered whether Alison held a broader assumption of which this was a subset—for example, "If I disappoint others, it means I'm bad." Upon questioning, though, the therapist determined that Alison did not generally place a special meaning on not accommodating her sister or others. The assumption she made about her sister was situation-specific and not linked to an important broader assumption. Having ascertained that the assumption was not part of a larger pattern, the therapist quickly moved on to discuss more central problems and cognitions.

THE COGNITIVE CONCEPTUALIZATION DIAGRAM

A Cognitive Conceptualization Diagram helps therapists organize the vast amount of data they obtain about and from patients. It helps them to:

- Identify patients' core beliefs, assumptions, and behavioral strategies.
- Understand why patients developed such extreme beliefs about themselves, others, and their worlds.
- Understand how patients' behavioral strategies are connected to their core beliefs.
- Determine which beliefs and behavioral strategies are most important to work on.
- Understand why patients currently react in a particular way: how their beliefs influence their perceptions of current situations and how these perceptions, in turn, influence their emotional, behavioral, and physiological reactions.

The Cognitive Conceptualization Diagram in Figure 2.1, for example, organizes much of the material already presented about Andrea and adds information about her childhood experiences that helps explain why she developed such extreme ideas about herself, others, and her world.

The bottom half of the diagram illustrates the cognitive model: in specific situations, patients have certain thoughts that influence their reactions. Therapists will find it useful to mentally fill out the boxes in the diagram from their first contact with a patient. However, it is best to start filling in the diagram (in pencil) after a few sessions, after having identified important patterns (1) in situations that lead to distress; (2) in patients' automatic thoughts; (3) in their emotional reactions; and (4) in their behavioral reactions. It is important to put a question mark next to any hypothesis not yet confirmed with the patient, since a hallmark in cognitive therapy is that conceptualizations are derived directly from the information that an individual patient provides.

When choosing problems/situations for the bottom of the diagram, the therapist looks for ones that are highly typical of the patient but that are different from one another—ones that exemplify different themes in the patient's automatic thoughts and different aspects of the patient's functioning and reactions. Choosing situations in which the automatic thoughts are too similar, for example, may lead the therapist to overlook important beliefs. On the other hand, choosing situations that are not typical of the patient will also lead to an inaccurate conceptualization.

The bottom of the diagram is actually an oversimplification. As described at the end of this chapter, patients may have many automatic thoughts associated with different emotions in a given situation. And patients may appraise their reactions (emotional, behavioral, and physiological) in a dysfunctional way. Also, patients frequently experience a *series* of thoughts before they engage in dysfunctional behaviors.

In addition, especially for patients with complex difficulties, three situations are too few—the therapist may need several (or many) more to fully capture patients' dysfunctional beliefs and strategies. It is also quite helpful to record situations in which the patient displays therapy-interfering behaviors, such as those described in Chapter 1. For example, if the therapist has not made a therapeutic error, it is useful to conceptualize the patient's thoughts that led to behaviors such as continually saying "I don't know," failing to follow through on homework, or talking in a hostile manner to the therapist. Figure 2.2 shows three situations in which Andrea displayed dysfunctional behavior in session. Note that the patient's conditional assumptions about therapy and the therapist are subsets of the broader assumptions in the Cognitive Conceptualization Diagram in Figure 2.1.

In completing the bottom part of the diagram, Andrea's therapist asks her for the *meaning* of her automatic thoughts. These meanings are

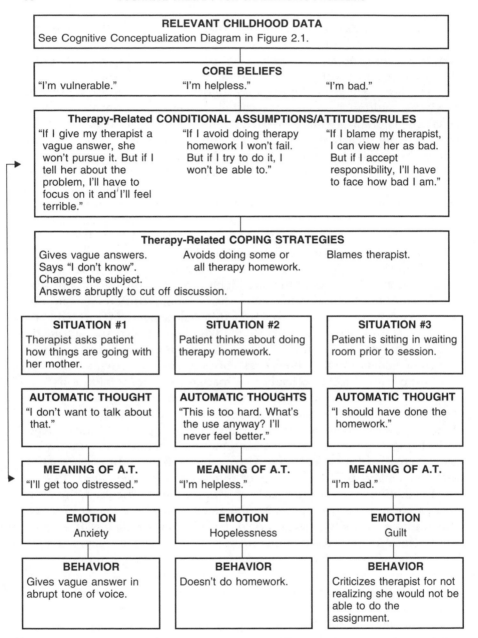

FIGURE 2.2. Cognitive Conceptualization Diagram illustrating therapy-interfering behaviors.

thematically linked to Andrea's core beliefs about the self, as shown in the top part of the diagram. In actuality, the patient's core beliefs act as a lens that affects Andrea's perceptions, and, as such, belong between the situation and the automatic thoughts. But in treatment, therapists generally elicit patients' beliefs by asking them for the meaning of their automatic thoughts. That is why the meaning box is placed below the automatic thought box. More properly, the box would appear above the automatic thought box and would be labeled "belief influencing the patient's perception of the situation."

In Andrea's case, she has believed since childhood that she is bad, helpless, and vulnerable. How did she develop these beliefs? The data presented in the top box make it clear why she began to see herself and others in such a negative light. She grew up in a chaotic and abusive household. At some point in treatment, her therapist will summarize Andrea's childhood experiences and help her see that many children who suffered the same kind of trauma she did might grow up with extreme beliefs about themselves and others—but that those beliefs might not be true, or not completely true.

Her therapist also helps her see that given these highly negative and dysfunctional beliefs, it would be natural for someone like Andrea to develop certain coping strategies to get along in the world. Andrea's therapist reviews her conditional assumptions so that Andrea can begin to understand why she often behaves so dysfunctionally. Andrea implicitly believes that if she uses her coping strategies, she will be okay, but if she does not use them, her core beliefs will become evident to herself or others.

THE COGNITIVE MODEL—ELABORATED

It is often important to elaborate upon the simplified cognitive model presented at the beginning of this chapter and in the Cognitive Conceptualization Diagram. Therapists and patients need to recognize that a range of situations (not all of which are discrete events) can trigger automatic thoughts. Moreover the sequence between triggering event and eventual behavior may be complex.

Situations/Triggers

Most people think of situations as discrete events, such as driving to therapy, having an argument with a partner, or opening an upsetting letter. But each component of the cognitive model may itself become a new trigger situation. Joel, for example, was feeling okay until the end of a phone call with his mother when he perceived that his mother was criticizing him for not calling her often enough (first situation). Joel thought, "Why does she always complain that I don't talk to her enough? Doesn't she know that I have a life?" He felt annoyed. Next Joel reflected on these thoughts (second situation) and had another set of thoughts, "I shouldn't think badly of Mom. She's old and lonely." Now he felt guilty. Then he noticed he was feeling guilty (third situation) and thought, "I'm a grown man. How come Mom still affects me so strongly? There's really something wrong with me." At this point he felt sad and sank down on the couch. Then he reflected on his behavior (fourth situation) and thought, "I shouldn't just sit here. What's the matter with me?" and he felt angry at himself.

Situations that trigger automatic thoughts may be:

- Discrete events
- Distressing thoughts
- Memories
- Images
- Emotions
- Behaviors
- Physiological sensations
- Mental sensations

In short, the situation part of the cognitive model can be any internal or external event or condition that people appraise in a personally meaningful way (see Figure 2.3).

When Automatic Thoughts Are Stimulus Situations

Automatic thoughts become situations when patients appraise them, that is, when patients become aware of their automatic thoughts and have additional automatic thoughts about them. Often the original automatic thoughts and the appraisals are verbal in form. For example, Bennett saw a homeless person sprawled out on the sidewalk, shouting obscenities (situation 1) and had the thought "This homeless person is disgusting." He became aware of this thought (situation 2) and appraised it: "I should never think things like that. I'm really rotten."

Automatic thoughts can also be imaginal in nature. Dena heard a noise (situation 1) and had an image of her baby falling down the stairs. She became aware of this image (situation 2) and appraised it: "Since I imagined [the baby falling down the stairs], I must want it to happen!"

When patients do appraise their thoughts, therapists need to conceptualize whether to focus on the original automatic thought or on its appraisal. Often the latter is significantly more important.

1. Single event: Therapist asks patient if she did the homework.
   ↓
   Automatic thought: "If I tell her I didn't do it, she'll get mad at me."

2. Distressing thoughts: Patient catches herself obsessing about germs.
   ↓
   Automatic thought: "There I go again. I must be crazy."

3. Memory: Patient has a spontaneous memory of being attacked.
   ↓
   Automatic thought: "I'm always going to be plagued by these flashbacks."

4. Image: Patient imagines her father crashing his car.
   ↓
   Automatic thought: "Oh, no! I must secretly want him to get hurt."

5. Emotion: Patient realizes that she is quite angry.
   ↓
   Automatic thought: "There is definitely something wrong with me. Normal people don't get this mad over something trivial."

6. Behavior: Patient has just purged.
   ↓
   Automatic thought: "I'm never going to get over my eating disorder."

7. Physiological sensation: Patient feels tightness in his chest.
   ↓
   Automatic thought: "I'm going to have a heart attack."

8. Mental experience: Patient recognizes his thoughts are racing.
   ↓
   Automatic thought: "I'm going crazy."

FIGURE 2.3. Examples of triggering situations.

When Reactions Are Stimulus Situations

Patients' reactions fall into three categories: emotional, behavioral, and physiological. It is important to ascertain if their reaction in and of itself is upsetting to them. Patients are often distressed by their *negative emotions*. Phil, for example, was in a drugstore (situation 1) and thought, "What if this medicine doesn't help me?" This thought made him feel quite anxious. Then he noticed how anxious he was feeling (situation 2) and thought, "My anxiety is never going to go away," and started to feel hopeless.

Sometimes patients are distressed by their *behavior*. Mary saw a plate of cookies at work (situation 1) and thought, "It will be okay to have just one," and took a cookie and ate it. When she finished eating, she realized what she had done (situation 2) and thought, "Oh, no, I shouldn't have eaten that. I've really blown my diet for the day. I might as well eat more and start again tomorrow."

Sometimes patients are most distressed by their *physiological reaction*. William, for example, was driving (situation 1), had automatic thoughts and images about crashing his car, felt anxious and realized his heart had started to beat quite rapidly. He noticed his heart beating rapidly (situation 2) and thought, "Oh, no, what's happening to me?" Patients' appraisals of their reactions may, in fact, be more important to focus on than the initial trigger situation.

Elaborated Sequences of the Cognitive Model

Having identified a problematic situation, therapists should determine whether there is an extended sequence of events, thoughts, and reactions—so that the therapist and patient can collaboratively decide where to start working. Often therapists must question patients carefully to determine their automatic thoughts before, during, and after a given situation. Doing so helps the therapist conceptualize where to focus:

- On the problem situation itself
- On one or more of the automatic thoughts about the situation
- On the dysfunctional beliefs that became activated
- On the patient's emotional reaction
- On the patient's behavior
- On the patient's appraisal of his/her thoughts, emotional reaction, or behavior

It is particularly important to draw an elaborated sequence when the patient becomes engaged in a dysfunctional cycle of thought–emotion–

behavior–physiological reaction as in a panic attack or when the patient engages in compulsive behavior such as substance abuse, bingeing and purging, violence toward others, or self-harming behavior.

Case Example 1

Maria always had a predictable sequence of events before and during a panic attack (though she and her therapist could not always identify the specific triggering event). A typical sequence was as follows (see Figure 2.4). Maria is riding in the car on the turnpike with her husband. She sees a sign and realizes that the nearest exit is far away. She thinks, "What if I get sick and need help?"

This thought leads Maria to feel quite anxious and her heart beats very quickly. She notices her rapid heartbeat and thinks "What's wrong with me?" She also pictures herself having a heart attack. She then feels significantly more anxious and her body reacts: her heart starts to pound, she breathes very quickly and deeply, and her chest starts to hurt. As she focuses on her physical reaction, her sensations intensify, and she begins to believe that she is about to have a heart attack. Her anxiety increases to panic, her body reacts (i.e., her sensations intensify), she focuses even more on her sensations, and she becomes increasingly convinced that she is having a heart attack.

The cycle continues for another 10 minutes until her body runs out of adrenaline and the sensations start to subside. After the panic attack, she thinks, "That was horrible. It'd better not happen again or next time I might really die." She feels anxious and her belief about her vulnerability becomes stronger.

Case Example 2

Patrick experiences a particular sequence of thoughts, sensations, and behaviors just prior to using drugs (see Figure 2.5). For example, he is at home, thinking about how little money he has, and feels sad. He realizes that he is feeling sad and thinks, "I hate this feeling. If only I could take a hit [of cocaine]." He then remembers the first time he took cocaine and how wonderful he felt. This image provokes craving and he feels an urge to use. He thinks, "I've got to get some. It won't hurt this one time." Patrick then actively makes a plan to get cocaine, focusing his attention on the plan and pushing away thoughts that might deter him. He then implements the plan, gets the cocaine, and snorts it. Hours later, he feels terrible again. His beliefs about being a failure and out of control intensify and predispose him to a greater lapse.

Situation 1: Patient realizes that she is far from a hospital.
↓

Activation of schema with belief "I'm vulnerable."
↓

Automatic thought: "What if I get sick and need help?"
↓

Emotion: Anxiety.
↓

Physiological reaction: Her heart beats faster.
↓

Situation 2: Patient realizes her heart is beating faster than normal.
↓

Automatic thought: "What's wrong with me?" Image of herself having a heart attack.
↓

Emotion: Anxiety intensifies.
↓

Physiological reaction: Her heart pounds, she hyperventilates, she becomes short of breath, and her chest hurts.
↓

Behavior and *Situation 3:* She focuses on her physical symptoms.
↓

Automatic thought: "I'm feeling worse and worse."
↓

Emotion: Her anxiety continues to intensify.
↓

Physiological reaction and *Situation 4:* Her symptoms intensify.
↓

Automatic thought: "I'm having a heart attack!"
↓

Emotion: Panic.
↓

Situation 5: Panic attack subsides.
↓

Automatic thought: "That was horrible. If it happens again, next time I might really die."
↓

Increase in belief of vulnerability.

FIGURE 2.4. Panic scenario.

Situation 1: Sitting at home.
↓

Automatic thought: "I'm so broke. I'll never get out of this hole."
↓

Emotion: Sad, hopeless.
↓

Situation 2: Notices feeling of sadness.
↓

Automatic thought: "I hate this feeling. If only I could take a hit [of cocaine]."
↓

Emotion: Anxious.
↓

Automatic thoughts: Memory of wonderful feeling he had the first time he tried cocaine.
↓

Emotion: Excited.
↓

Physiological reaction: Craving.
↓

Situation 3: Recognizes uncomfortable cravings.
↓

Automatic thought: "I've got to get some [cocaine]. It won't hurt this one time."
↓

Emotion: Relief.
↓

Behavior: Pushes away thoughts that could deter him; gets cocaine, snorts it.
↓

Situation 4: Hours later, realizes what he's done.
↓

Automatic thought: "I can't believe I did that. I'm so weak. I'll never beat this [addiction]."
↓

Increase in beliefs of being a failure and out of control.

FIGURE 2.5. Substance use scenario.

Case Example 3

Pamela has bulimia. Her pattern of bingeing is typical (see Figure 2.6). Having finished the late shift at the factory where she works, she comes home to an empty apartment and feels at loose ends. "I should probably do my laundry," she thinks, "but I don't really feel like it." She starts thinking about her family and friends, all of whom live more than an hour away. She realizes how lonely she is and thinks, "I can't stand this [distress]! What can I do?" She tries to read a magazine but can't concentrate. She thinks, "Food will calm me down. I know I ate enough today, but I'm too upset. I can't help it."

Pamela remembers that there is ice cream in the freezer. She has a visual image and a somatic sensation of eating the ice cream that is quite pleasurable. This image triggers craving and Pamela experiences a strong urge to get the ice cream and start eating. She overrides her thoughts that discourage her from going to the freezer and makes the decision that she is going to eat. Having made this decision, she experiences relief. She takes the quart of ice cream out of the freezer and starts to eat it. She tells herself she will stop after a few bites. After several spoonfuls she thinks, "I know I should stop, but I'm still too upset," and continues eating. She pushes away the thoughts that might regulate her behavior; in fact, she tries to clear her mind of all thoughts. Almost in a dissociative state, she continues to eat and eat until all the ice cream is gone. Then she looks around for more food. After finishing the binge, she feels physically and emotionally terrible. She has a highly exaggerated image of herself as bloated and obese. She blames herself viciously for being so weak and out of control. Her dysphoria deepens and she gives herself permission to purge.

SUMMARY

Patients tend to think and behave in consistent ways, in accordance with their beliefs and coping strategies. It is essential to continually refine a cognitive conceptualization to help understand why patients react in the ways they do to current situations and to select the most important problems, cognitions, and behaviors on which to focus. Part of the art of cognitive therapy lies in developing accurate conceptualizations, particularly when patients' difficulties are quite complex, and in using those conceptualizations to guide treatment. The next chapter, which describes the cognitive formulation of personality disorders, can help the clinician to more quickly identify the underpinnings of their Axis II patients' historical and current difficulties.

Situation 1: Home alone in the evening.
↓
Automatic thought: "I should do my laundry, but I don't feel like it. I wish I were with [my family and friends]."
↓
Emotion: Lonely.
↓
Situation 2: Notices she is feeling quite lonely.
↓
Automatic thought: "I can't stand this. What can I do?"
↓
Emotion: Anxious.
↓
Automatic thought: "The only thing that will make me feel better is food."
↓
Image of eating ice cream.
↓
Physiological reaction: Craving.
↓
Automatic thought: "I know I shouldn't, but I'm going to go get it."
↓
Emotion: Relief.
↓
Behavior: Gets ice cream. Eats several tablespoons.
↓
Automatic thought: "I should stop. But I'm still too upset."
↓
Behavior: Pushes away thoughts. Finishes the carton. Continues to eat other high-carbohydrate, high-fat food.
↓
Situation: Feels physically unwell.
↓
Automatic thoughts and image: "I'm so stupid. I should never have done that." [Image of self as grossly bloated and fat.]
↓
Emotion: Sad, hopeless, angry at self.
↓
Automatic thought: "I can't stand this. I have to make myself vomit."
↓
Emotion: Partial relief.
↓
Behavior: Purges.
↓
Increase in beliefs that she is bad, undesirable, and out of control.

FIGURE 2.6. Scenario of bulimia.

CHAPTER 3

███████

When a Personality Disorder Challenges Treatment

Although not all patients who present challenges in treatment have under-lying personality disorders, many do. Therefore it is helpful to the clini-cian to understand the cognitive formulation for each Axis II disorder. The DSM-IV-TR (American Psychiatric Association, 2000) thoroughly cov-ers the affective and behavioral symptoms present in the various mental disorders, including personality disorders. However, the cognitive aspects of these disorders are not given nearly as much attention, even though cognitive factors are important for their assessment and treatment. Recent data suggest each personality disorder has a specific set of associated beliefs (Beck et al., 2001). Understanding what these cognitions are for each Axis II disorder aids therapists in quickly conceptualizing patients' problems and deciding how to intervene most effectively.

Therapists can also use this understanding to diagnose therapeutic relationship problems on the spot and to modify the structure, style, and interventions they are using as needed. Of course, most patients do not have traits from just one Axis II disorder: they often display a mixture of beliefs and strategies. However, the examples in this chapter can be a use-ful guide when therapists are trying to make sense of the bewildering array of cognitions, behaviors, and emotional reactions of patients with personality disorders.

This chapter explains how individuals develop personality disorders. It outlines, for each Axis II disorder, patients' beliefs about the self and others, their conditional assumptions, their overdeveloped and underde-veloped strategies, and their specific beliefs and behaviors that can inter-fere with treatment. A case example is also presented for each personality disorder. Chapter 10 describes how to elicit patients' beliefs and Appendix B presents the Personality Belief Questionnaire (Beck & J. Beck, 1995), which can be used to identify and categorize beliefs from each Axis II disorder. For a comprehensive account of the categorization, theory, assessment, and treatments for personality disorders, see Millon (1996). For an extensive description of the application of cognitive therapy to personality disorders, see Beck et al. (2004).

HOW DO PEOPLE DEVELOP PERSONALITY DISORDERS?

Cognitive therapists view the development of Axis II disorders as the result of an interaction between individuals' genetic predispositions toward certain personality traits and their early experiences. A histrionic patient, for example, may have been born with a flair for the dramatic. A schizoid patient may have a disposition toward preferring isolation to social contact. A narcissistic patient may have a strong bent toward competitiveness. The meaning children make out of their childhood experiences—especially overtly traumatic events or more subtle, but very negative and chronic experiences—may increase the expression of these inherited tendencies.

Case Example

Kate was quite shy, awkward, and sensitive by nature. As a child, she was often teased by her peers and criticized by her parents. She started to believe that there was something wrong with her—that she was basically unlikable or unacceptable. These ideas were quite painful to her, so she tried to avoid their activation. Kate became very meek in interactions with her parents and other authority figures, and tried to avoid attracting their attention, which she predicted was likely to be negative. She began to limit contact with her classmates and children in the neighborhood, fearing that if she approached them they would be mean to her.

Kate's meekness provoked additional criticism from her parents, which in turn increased her beliefs of being defective. When she withdrew further from other children, they began to ignore her completely, which in turn increased her belief that she was unlikable. (Her limited social contact with other children also prevented her from developing the social skills that other children learned through repeated social interactions with peers.) Her avoidant behaviors increased the strength of her beliefs, which led to her engaging in these behaviors even more, which continued to strengthen her beliefs, in a continuous negative cycle.

Kate also seemed prewired to experience negative emotions more intensely than others. She developed a belief that she was vulnerable to distressing feelings, assuming she would "fall apart" if they increased in intensity. She developed dysfunctional ways to deal with her negative emotions by avoiding social contact, avoiding thinking about distressing things, and distracting herself.

If Kate continues to use avoidance as a major strategy, if she fails to develop more functional ways to cope with her negative emotions, and if her core beliefs that she is unlovable and unacceptable grow stronger, she may be at risk of developing avoidant personality disorder.

Patients may also be *positively* reinforced for their strategies or they may model themselves after others. Jay's father had strong obsessive–compulsive traits. As a child, Jay continually observed his father's perfectionistic, overcontrolling behavior. In addition, his father praised Jay for keeping his room extremely neat and for getting straight A's in school (and disapproved of Jay's less organized, more unruly siblings). Jay developed rigid beliefs about the utter necessity of orderliness, self-control, high standards, and perfectionism that amplified his natural behavioral tendencies in these areas.

TYPICAL OVERDEVELOPED AND UNDERDEVELOPED STRATEGIES

Patients with personality disorders are characterized by having a relatively small set of behavioral strategies that they use across situations and across time, even when these strategies are clearly dysfunctional (Beck et al., 2004). They develop these strategies as a way to cope with their highly negative core beliefs. Before treatment, most Axis II patients do not have a great deal of choice in the coping behaviors they employ. They simply do not learn a wide array of strategies, and therefore lack a sufficient repertoire of behaviors from which to select according to the context (J. Beck, 1997).

Therapeutically, it is critical to view strategies people employ as neither "good" nor "bad." Rather, they are either more or less *adaptive* according to the situation and their goals. People with healthy personalities are able to use a variety of strategies effectively. For example, it is useful for people to be hypervigilant when they are walking in a dangerous part of town, to depend on their family and friends when they are sick, to be competitive when they are trying to advance their careers, to be detail-oriented when they are doing their taxes. It is not adaptive for people to be paranoid around their trustworthy friends, to be overly dependent on partners to make them feel better, to compete with their children, or to be unnecessarily dramatic during a medical emergency.

There are a small number of overdeveloped strategies specific to each personality disorder (Beck et al., 2004; Pretzer & Beck, 1996), as outlined below. These strategies may or may not have been relatively adaptive when they were first developed, but they invariably lead to significant difficulty later on when individuals use these behaviors compulsively and are unable to use other approaches that are more adaptive to the situation. Patients often use these strategies both outside of therapy and also in the therapy session itself. For example, a patient who is hypervigilant for harm from others may well be suspicious of his or her therapist as well.

These characteristic coping strategies can pose difficulties for therapists. When patients display dysfunctional behavior in session, therapists should realize that their patients' behaviors likely stem from difficult (often traumatic) life circumstances and extreme, negative core beliefs. Such a stance allows therapists to regard patients more positively, display empathy, and behave more adaptively themselves.

It is essential for therapists to assess the range and rigidity of patients' strategies as part of their overall conceptualization in order to develop realistic expectations and to guide their treatment. It would be unreasonable, for example, to expect a patient with narcissistic personality disorder to suddenly stop acting superior and demanding at the beginning of therapy. A patient with strong passive–aggressive features is unlikely to be able to carry out standard homework assignments early in treatment.

Failure to recognize patients' underdeveloped skills could lead therapists to encourage them to make changes before they have developed the requisite skill to do so. As illustrated below, this kind of therapeutic error can have significant consequences.

Case Example

Maggie was a 19-year-old woman with moderate depression and dependent and avoidant personality disorders. She lived with her parents. Her therapist accurately conceptualized that Maggie's depression was exacerbated by her parents' frequent criticism of her. When the therapist learned that her older sister, Jen, was more positive and supportive and willing to take her in, he suggested that Maggie move to Jen's house.

While Jen herself was warmer and more positive, Jen's husband was more intrusive and kept insisting that Maggie take on new challenges, such as going out with peers, looking for a better job, and taking care of her own finances. Maggie was ill equipped to deal with these activities. She lacked the capacity at that point to make decisions, solve problems, initiate conversations (much less new relationships), handle her finances, and tolerate negative emotion.

Unable to cope with these demands, Maggie became more and more anxious. Her beliefs of incompetence and worthlessness became greatly activated and her depression worsened significantly. She started to feel quite hopeless about ever being able to lead a happy, normal life and began, for the first time, to seriously consider the possibility of suicide.

COGNITIVE PROFILES OF SPECIFIC AXIS II DISORDERS

Each personality disorder is listed below, in order of its prevalence in community samples (Torgersen, Kringlen, & Cramer, 2001), along with its corresponding set of beliefs (about the self and others), assumptions, over and underdeveloped strategies, and therapy-interfering cognitions and behaviors. Each personality disorder is also illustrated by a specific case example.

Histrionic Personality Disorder

Beliefs about the Self

"I am nothing" (activated when others are inattentive or disapproving). (Also, "I am wonderful, special" [activated when others display a positive reaction toward the patient].)

Beliefs about Others

"I need to impress others to get their caring."

Conditional Assumptions

"If I entertain others, they'll like me (but if I don't, they'll ignore me)."
"If I'm dramatic, I'll get my needs met (but if I'm not, I won't get what I need from other people)."

Overdeveloped Coping Strategies

Being overly dramatic.
Dressing, acting, speaking seductively.
Entertaining others.
Seeking adulation.

Underdeveloped Coping Strategies

Being quiet, submissive.
Blending in with others.
Holding reasonable standards for others' behavior toward the patient.
Valuing acting within normal limits.

Therapy-Interfering Beliefs

"If I entertain my therapist, she will like me."
"If I dramatize my problems, my therapist will want to help me."
"If I act 'normally' in treatment, I'll be 'average' and boring."

Therapy-Interfering Behaviors

Creating a dramatic appearance.
Speaking entertainingly.
Acting seductively.
Soliciting adulation.
Avoiding homework assignments that lead the patient to feel ordinary.

Case Example

As a young child, Tiffany was the center of her parents' and grandparents' lives. She was highly engaging and outgoing. She loved entertaining others. But the intensely positive attention, recognition, and special treatment she received diminished almost overnight at age 8 when her brother was born with significant health problems. Her parents, burdened with the care of a very sick baby, criticized her for demanding attention. Tiffany went from believing that she was the most special, precious little girl in the world to believing that she was "nothing."

The sense of emotional deprivation and being disregarded was quite painful to Tiffany, so she developed strategies to try to recapture her sense of being special. She began to try to elicit the interest of others whenever she could, through dramatic language and emotional reactions, artistic endeavors such as singing and acting in school plays, and several years later through dressing and speaking in a very seductive manner and entering beauty contests. She believed that she could only be happy if others took notice of her and treated her specially. Tiffany also tended to experience emotions more intensely than others. Compared to many people, she felt higher "highs" when praised or doted on but much lower "lows" when she was not.

When she first entered treatment, Tiffany tried to use her usual strategies, entertaining her therapist, regaling her with stories minimally related to her actual problems, and bringing her gifts.

Obsessive–Compulsive Personality Disorder

Beliefs about the Self

"I am vulnerable to bad things happening."
"I am responsible for preventing harm."

Beliefs about Others

"Other people are weak, irresponsible, careless."

Conditional Assumptions

"If I take responsibility for everything, I'll be okay (but if I depend on others, they'll let me down)."

"If I create and maintain order for myself and others and do everything perfectly, my world will be okay (but if I don't, everything will fall apart)."

Overdeveloped Coping Strategies

Rigidly controlling self and others.
Creating unreasonable expectations.
Assuming too much responsibility.
Striving for perfection.

Underdeveloped Coping Strategies

Delegating authority.
Developing flexible expectations.
Exercising control only when appropriate.
Tolerating uncertainty.
Acting spontaneously and impulsively.
Seeking fun and pleasurable activities.

Therapy-Interfering Beliefs

"If I don't correct my therapist and tell her exactly what she needs to know, she won't be able to help me."

"If I don't do my therapy assignments perfectly, therapy won't work."

"If I lower my expectations for myself and others, bad things will happen."

Therapy-Interfering Behaviors

Trying to control the session.
Trying to impart perfectly correct information.
Being hypervigilant for therapist's lack of understanding.
Spending excessive time and care on homework.
Resisting assignments to be spontaneous and delegate responsibility.

Case Example

Dennis was the oldest of five children whose parents were alcoholics. From a young age, Dennis felt vulnerable. He saw others as unpredictable and irresponsible. His world seemed chaotic. Dennis soon learned that if he took on an adult role, his world felt somewhat safer. It became quite adaptive for Dennis to keep his emotions in check, to develop rules and systems to create order in the household, and to be overly responsible for himself and his younger siblings.

These strategies also served him well as an adult in his work life, as a self-employed computer programmer. Unfortunately, though, he was never able to develop healthy relationships with women. The strategies that served him so well as a child and later in his work became highly ingrained and Dennis never learned counterbalancing strategies: how to delegate responsibility, how to be flexible in his expectations and rules for himself and others, how to be lighthearted and impulsive, how to have fun. Women invariably found him to be too serious, overly responsible, rigid, and perfectionistic.

His therapist soon found that Dennis' obsessive–compulsive traits also interfered with treatment. Dennis tried to control the therapy session, overriding his therapist's gentle efforts to interrupt. He provided overly detailed accounts of his difficulties so that his therapist could understand him perfectly. And he tried to be overly perfectionist when he did his therapy homework.

Passive–Aggressive Personality Disorder[1]

Beliefs about the Self

"I am vulnerable to being controlled by others."
"I am misunderstood and unappreciated."

Beliefs about Others

"Other people are strong, intrusive, demanding."
"They have unreasonable expectations of me."
"They should leave me alone."

Conditional Assumptions

"If others control me, it means I'm weak."
"If I exert indirect control (e.g., by agreeing outwardly but not following

---

[1]From DSM-III-R (American Psychiatric Association, 1987).

through), others will be unable to control me (but if I assert myself directly, it won't work)."

Overdeveloped Coping Strategies

Pretending to cooperate.
Avoiding assertion, confrontation, and direct refusal.
Resisting others' control passively.
Resisting taking on responsibility.
Resisting fulfilling others' expectations.

Underdeveloped Coping Strategies

Cooperating.
Assuming reasonable responsibility for self and others.
Doing straightforward interpersonal problem solving.

Therapy-Interfering Beliefs

"If I do what my therapist asks, it means she's in control and I'm weak."
"If I assert myself directly with my therapist, she'll exert more control."
"If I improve through therapy, other people will expect too much of me."

Therapy-Interfering Behaviors

Collaboratively setting homework assignments but failing to follow
    through.
Remaining passive during problem solving.
Outwardly agreeing with what therapist says but privately disagreeing.

Case Example

Claire was hypersensitive to control even when she was in elementary school. She was quite bothered when authority figures (e.g., her parents, teachers, other adults) told her what to do, especially if she perceived the task as difficult or unpleasant. Ironically, she later married (because she had become pregnant) a man who was somewhat overcontrolling. When he gave her lists of tasks to do (balancing the checkbook, using coupons at the grocery store, reorganizing closets at home), she would promise to do them, but rarely followed through. When he disciplined their son, she found ways to undermine his authority with the child. Claire found it relatively easy to secure part-time jobs but had a history of lasting only weeks or months before she was let go because she failed to live up to her bosses' expectations.

Claire's beliefs that she was weak and likely to be controlled became activated in therapy and she displayed her characteristic behaviors, agreeing, for example, to do homework assignments but then not following through. She continually confirmed her therapist's hypotheses, whether or not she really agreed with them.

Borderline Personality Disorder

Beliefs about the Self

"I am bad, worthless."
"I am unlovable, defective."
"I am helpless, out of control."
"I am incompetent."
"I am weak and vulnerable."
"I am a victim."

Beliefs about Others

"Others are strong."
"Others are potentially hurtful."
"Others are superior."
"Others will reject and abandon me."

Conditional Assumptions

"If I avoid challenges, I'll be okay (but if I take on challenges, I'll fail)."
"If I depend on others, I'll be okay (but if I don't, I won't survive)."
"If I do everything others want, they may stay with me for the time being (but if I displease them, they'll abandon me sooner)."
"If I'm hypervigilant for harm from other people, I can protect myself (but if I'm not, I'll get hurt)."
"If I punish others when I'm upset, I can feel more powerful and perhaps control their future behavior (but if I don't, I'll feel weak and they may hurt me again)."
"If I cut off my negative emotions, I'll be okay (but if I don't, I'll fall apart)."

Overdeveloped Coping Strategies

Mistrusting others.
Blaming others.
Avoiding challenges.
Depending on others.

Overly subjugating self to or dominating others.
Avoiding negative emotion.
Self harming when emotions are intense.

Underdeveloped Coping Strategies

Balancing one's needs against another's.
Looking for nonmalignant explanations for others' behavior.
Trusting others.
Calming self down.
Solving interpersonal problems.
Persisting in difficult activities.

Therapy-Interfering Beliefs

"I can get better and survive only if I completely depend on my therapist."
"If I trust my therapist, she'll end up rejecting and abandoning me, so I might as well reject her first."
"If I focus on solving problems, it won't work and I'll end up feeling worse."

Therapy-Interfering Behaviors

Disparaging the therapist.
Overly relying on the therapist to feel better.
Making too many crisis calls between sessions.
Demanding entitlements from the therapist.

Case Example

June's mother died when June was 6 years old. Naturally, she felt devastated. She had no one to turn to after her mother's death, and never quite recovered from this loss. Her father was both neglectful and emotionally abusive to her. She began to believe her father when he repeatedly told her she was bad and worthless. She became highly fearful, expecting that her father would continue to hurt her or might abandon her; she also expected that other people would do the same. June was relatively noncommunicative and isolative both at home and at school. She rejected help from teachers and neighbors when they reached out to her. As an adolescent, June developed friendships for the first time, but with undependable teens who used drugs and enjoyed being "counterculture" in their speech, dress, and general mien. She became angrier and angrier at her father and, with the support of her friends, became a frequent runaway.

When June entered treatment for substance abuse and depression, she believed that her therapist would harm her. Indeed, she had previously been hurt in therapy when a therapist took advantage of her vulnerability and sexually seduced her. She feared that her current therapist would lie to her and manipulate her, too. On the other hand, June soon became highly dependent on her therapist, believing that he was her only lifeline. She became quite angry when he tried to place reasonable limits on contact with her outside of the session and when he tried to end sessions on time. She accused him of not caring about her and started to show up late for sessions.

Dependent Personality Disorder

Beliefs about the Self

"I am incompetent."
"I am weak."
"I need others to survive."

Beliefs about Others

"Others are strong and capable."

Conditional Assumptions

"If I depend on others, I'll be okay (but if I depend on myself—make decisions, try to solve problems—I'll fail)."
"If I subjugate myself to others, they'll take care of me (but If I upset them, they won't)."

Overdeveloped Coping Strategies

Relying on others.
Avoiding making decisions.
Avoiding solving problems independently.
Trying to keep others happy.
Subjugating self to others.
Being meek and submissive.

Underdeveloped Coping Strategies

Solving problems independently.
Making decisions.
Asserting self with others.

Therapy-Interfering Beliefs

"If I try to use my skills independently, I'll fail."
"If I practice assertion, I'll alienate others."
"If I terminate therapy, I won't be able to handle life."

Therapy-Interfering Behaviors

Looking to the therapist to solve the patient's problems and make decisions for him/her.
Trying too hard to please the therapist.
Resisting homework assignments involving assertion.

Case Example

Sheila was a clingy, and fearful child. Even when asked to do tasks that she was capable of performing, she frequently felt overwhelmed and confused and asked for far more help than she really needed. Eventually she began to see herself as wholly incompetent. Her mother, perceiving her daughter as somewhat backward, allowed Sheila to rely heavily on her and did not encourage independence. Sheila became skilled at asking others for help, requesting that others make decisions for her, and avoiding conflict. She learned that if she subjugated her desires to others, they would allow her to cling to them.

Sheila was able to use these strategies effectively while she was still living with her widowed mother. When her mother remarried, however, her stepfather insisted that Sheila, now 21, move out of the house in which she had grown up. She did not know how to fend for herself, make decisions, be assertive. She had to find a job to pay her bills. She grew increasingly anxious and developed generalized anxiety disorder.

Although her dependent features initially led her to be quite compliant in therapy (i.e., she was eager to please her therapist), Sheila had much difficulty taking the lead in solving problems and was fearful of terminating with her therapist, even after her anxiety disorder had remitted.

Avoidant Personality Disorder

Beliefs about the Self

"I'm unlovable, unacceptable, defective, bad."
"I'm vulnerable to negative emotion."

Beliefs about Others

"Others are superior, potentially critical, and rejecting."

Conditional Assumptions

"If I pretend I'm okay, others may accept me (but if I show my real self, they will reject me)."

"If I please others all the time, I'll be okay (but if I upset them, they'll hurt me)."

"If I (cognitively and behaviorally) avoid, I'll be okay (but if I allow myself to feel negative emotions, I'll fall apart)."

Overdeveloped Coping Strategies

Avoiding social situations.
Avoiding calling attention to self.
Avoiding revealing self to others.
Distrusting others.
Avoiding experiencing negative emotion.

Underdeveloped Coping Strategies

Approaching others.
Trusting others' positive motives.
Acting naturally around others.
Seeking intimacy.
Thinking about upsetting situations and problems.

Therapy-Interfering Beliefs

"If I trust my therapist's apparent care and compassion, I'll get hurt."
"If I focus on problems in therapy, I'll feel too overwhelmed."
"If I reveal negative parts of my history and current experience, my therapist will judge me negatively."
"If I try to work toward achieving interpersonal goals, I'll be rejected."
"If I assert myself reasonably, people won't like me."

Therapy-Interfering Behaviors

Putting on a false front to therapist.
Avoiding revealing self.
Changing the subject when feeling distressed in the session.
Resisting homework assignments that could lead to distress.

Case Example

Erin grew up in difficult circumstances. Her father abandoned the family when Erin was just a toddler. Throughout Erin's childhood, she was continually blamed by her mother for his leaving. Her mother was cold and demeaning. Erin began to see herself as unlovable and unworthy. She assumed that if people really knew her, they would be critical and rejecting because she was so unlovable. She believed that she would never get the love and intimacy she so much wanted if she showed her true self to others.

Erin developed a strategy of avoidance. She avoided social situations whenever she could: she avoided talking to others at school, she avoided speaking up in class, she avoided calling attention to herself, she avoided revealing much about herself to anyone. She was also hypervigilant for others' negative evaluation of her—and frequently misperceived their neutral reactions as significantly negative.

Erin also felt very vulnerable to unpleasant emotion. She feared that if she allowed herself to experience deep dysphoria, she would fall apart. So she also avoided negative emotion, not only by avoiding potentially upsetting situations, but also by avoiding even *thinking* about distressing things. She also found that alcohol helped ease the pain of loneliness and depression. Her strategies of cognitive, emotional, and interpersonal avoidance contributed to difficulties in treatment when she entered therapy as a young adult for alcohol dependence.

Paranoid Personality Disorder

Beliefs about the Self

"I am weak and vulnerable (and must be on guard and/or take preemptive aggressive actions)."

Beliefs about Others

"Other people will hurt me."

Conditional Assumptions

"If I'm hypervigilant, I can pick up signs of [interpersonal] danger (but if I'm not on guard, I won't see them)."
"If I assume others are untrustworthy, I'll be able to protect myself (but if I trust others, they'll hurt me)."

Overdeveloped Coping Strategies

Being hypervigilant for harm.
Trusting no one.
Assuming hidden motives.
Expecting to be manipulated, taken advantage of, diminished.

Underdeveloped Coping Strategies

Trusting others.
Relaxing.
Cooperating.
Assuming good intentions.

Therapy-Interfering Beliefs

"If I trust my therapist, she'll hurt me."
"If I'm not on my guard in therapy, I'll be harmed."

Therapy-Interfering Behaviors

Rejecting signs of caring from the therapist.
Reject alternative explanations for others' behavior.
Resisting homework assignments to be more intimate with others.

Case Example

Jon developed a strategy of being hypervigilant for harm as he was growing up. Starting at age 3, he lived in a series of foster homes in which some of his foster parents were physically and emotionally abusive. He saw himself as vulnerable to people. In fact, it was quite adaptive for him in certain situations to be suspicious of others' motives and untrusting of their words. Unfortunately, Jon began to see *everyone* as potentially harmful. He was largely unable to discriminate between people who were likely to hurt him and those who were not.

Jon developed bipolar disorder in his early 20s. When he entered cognitive therapy treatment in his early 40s, he was quite distrustful of his therapist. He was noncompliant with medication, he refused to reveal much about himself, he was evasive in his answers to basic questions, and he was reluctant to monitor his thoughts, mood, and behavior. He assumed that if he trusted his therapist, she would harm him.

Antisocial Personality Disorder

Beliefs about the Self

"I am a potential victim (so my only viable alternative is to be a victimizer)."
" 'Normal' rules don't apply to me."

Beliefs about Others

"Others will try to control, manipulate, or take advantage of me."
"Others are there for me to exploit."

Conditional Assumptions

"If I manipulate or attack others first, I'll be on top (but if I don't, they could squash me)."

"If I act hostile and strong, I can do what I want (but if I don't, others will try to control me)."

Overdeveloped Coping Strategies

Lying.
Manipulating or taking advantage of others.
Threatening or attacking others.
Resisting others' control.
Acting impulsively.

Underdeveloped Coping Strategies

Cooperating with others.
Following societal rules.
Thinking about consequences.

Therapy-Interfering Beliefs

"If I dominate my therapist, she won't be able to control me."
"If I comply with my therapist, it will mean she is strong and I am weak."
"If I tell the truth, she will impose negative consequences."
"If I engage in treatment, I won't be able to do what I want."

Therapy-Interfering Behaviors

Trying to intimidate the therapist.
Lying to the therapist.
Trying to manipulate the therapist.
Engaging only superficially, if at all.

Case Example

Mickey grew up in a dysfunctional family. His mother was drug-dependent and alternated between neglecting and physically abusing her children. As a young child, Mickey was very anxious. He felt weak and vulnerable. At age 8, he discovered that beating up his younger brother could make him feel strong and superior. Then he began to prey on the weaker children in the neighborhood. He developed a drug habit at age 12. He and a group of friends engaged in petty thievery and purse snatching. By age 14, Mickey worked for drug dealers and later became a drug dealer himself.

Mickey emphatically did not want to be in treatment. A condition of his parole (he had been convicted of selling drugs) was to enter treatment or go to jail. Initially he lied to his therapist (especially about his drug use and thievery), came late to sessions, and seemed only superficially engaged.

Schizotypal Personality Disorder

Beliefs about the Self

"I am different."
"I have special powers."
"I am vulnerable."

Beliefs about Others

"Others won't understand me."
"Others will reject me."
"Others will hurt me."

Conditional Assumptions

"If I pursue 'unusual' interests such as the occult, I'll be different in a special way (but if I don't, I'll just be different in a defective way)."
"If I'm hypervigilant for harm, I can protect myself from others (but if I'm not, I'll get hurt)."
"If I distance myself from others, I'll be okay (but if I get close to people, they will hurt me)."

Overdeveloped Coping Strategies

Pursuing eccentric interests.
Being suspicious of others.
Distancing self from others.

Underdeveloped Coping Strategies

Trusting others.
Seeking out interactions with others.
Seeking rational explanations for unusual experiences.

Therapy-Interfering Beliefs

"If I trust my therapist, she'll hurt me."
"If my 'sixth sense' tells me something is true, it must be true."

Therapy-Interfering Behaviors

Resisting alternative explanations of events.
Avoiding fully revealing self to the therapist.
Looking for signs of harm from the therapist.

Case Example

Hank had always seemed strange to others. Even as a child, he looked odd. Other kids at school and in the neighborhood taunted and ridiculed him, leading him to develop a belief that he was different. This belief led him to withdraw from others. As an adolescent, Hank was drawn to the occult. He believed he had a "sixth sense" and favored wearing a cape. He became preoccupied with divining the future, reading special meanings into many everyday occurrences. He had no real friends and most of his social interaction was through the Internet, contacting others who were also interested in the occult through chat rooms and e-mail. Other people continued to shun him for his eccentricities. This rejection, combined with his self-imposed isolation, meant that Hank did not experience normal interaction with others and did not have opportunities to develop appropriate social skills.

Hank posed a challenge in therapy. He was chronically anxious and dysphoric but was fearful of setting goals to engage in activities that could improve his life, particularly those that might bring him into contact with other people. He felt quite vulnerable and at the beginning of treatment was continually suspicious of his therapist, believing that she might harm him.

Schizoid Personality Disorder

Beliefs about the Self

"I am different, defective; I don't fit in."

Beliefs about Others

"Others don't like me."
"Others are intrusive."

Conditional Assumptions

"If I keep to myself, others won't bother me (but if I engage with them, they'll find me lacking)."
"If I avoid relationships, I'll be okay (but if I get involved with others, they'll be too intrusive)."

Overdeveloped Coping Strategies

Avoiding contact with others.
Shunning intimacy.
Engaging in solitary pursuits.

Underdeveloped Coping Strategies

Possessing ordinary social skills.
Trusting others.

Therapy-Interfering Beliefs

"If my therapist displays caring and empathy, I'll feel too uncomfortable."
"If I set goals, I'll have to change my [isolated] life and I'll feel worse."

Therapy-Interfering Behaviors

Speaking little, avoiding self-disclosure.
Avoiding setting goals to improve the patient's life.
Resisting homework assignments involving interpersonal contact.

Case Example

Lee had always been a loner. Characterized as a "misfit" by his family, teachers, and peers, Lee rarely, if ever, sought out purely social contact. He seemed not to feel the psychic rewards of social interaction as most children and adults do. His behavioral strategy of avoidance helped him avoid the feelings of anxiety that invariably arose when he interacted with others. He was far more comfortable in solitary pursuits: building models, playing computer games, watching television. He was not terribly unhappy as a child but did feel different and somewhat defective.

As a young adult, Lee moved away from home and took jobs, such as a night security guard, that did not involve much contact with others. He became increasingly cognizant that his desire for human interaction and relationships was much lower than most people's—in fact, it was almost nil. He felt increasingly empty and unable to experience much of a sense of mastery or pleasure. His life continued to revolve around work and solitary activities.

When Lee entered treatment for depression, he had difficulty setting goals. Despite his dysphoria, his only objective was to get his mother "off my back," as she was continually hounding him to get a better job and find a circle of friends. He became anxious in therapy when his therapist demonstrated a caring, empathic attitude and when he perceived her as intrusive, asking too many questions about his thoughts and emotions.

Narcissistic Personality Disorder

Beliefs about the Self

"I am inferior, nothing, a piece of garbage" (activated when perceiving that others are disregarding or critical of the patient).
(Also, "I am superior" [activated when receiving special treatment or accolades from others].)

Beliefs about Others

"Others are superior, hurtful, demeaning."
(Also, "Others are inferior" [activated when perceiving others as less successful than the patient].)

Conditional Assumptions

"If I act in a superior way, I can feel better about myself (but if I don't, I'll feel painfully inferior)."
"If people treat me in special ways, it shows I am superior (but if they don't, I should punish them)."
"If I control others/put them down, I can feel superior to them (but if I don't, they'll put me down and make me feel inferior)."

Overdeveloped Coping Strategies

Demanding special treatment from others.
Being hypervigilant for shabby (or "normal") treatment from others.
Punishing others when feeling slighted, diminished, dysphoric.
Criticizing, putting people down, trying to compete with and control them.
Trying to impress people with material possessions, accomplishments, and intimacy with high-status people.

Underdeveloped Coping Strategies

Cooperating with others toward achieving a common goal.
Working diligently step by step to achieve personal goals.
Tolerating inconveniences, frustration, lack of recognition.
Meeting others' expectations without great benefit to self.

Therapy-Interfering Beliefs

"If I'm not vigilant, my therapist will put me down."

"If I don't impress her with my superiority, my therapist will think I'm inferior."

"If I don't punish my therapist for making me feel small, she'll do it again and again."

"If I don't push hard, I won't be treated in a special way."

Therapy-Interfering Behaviors

Trying to impress the therapist.

Demanding entitlements.

Treating the therapist as an inferior.

Punishing the therapist (through criticism, snide remarks) when feeling slighted.

Resisting agreeing to homework assignments the therapist suggests.

Case Example

Brad's father had a significantly negative impact on his son as he grew up. Highly narcissistic, his father continually pointed out his own accomplishments, demanded to be waited on hand and foot, and was quite critical of Brad for not being "a chip off the old block." While Brad was bright enough, he could never live up to his father's standards and developed a belief of worthlessness. He soon learned to mimic his father's behavior around other people, though, and felt better when he could convince himself and others that he was actually superior to them. He continually bragged about himself, demanded entitlements, and focused on others' weaknesses. On the other hand, he was hypersensitive and reacted quite strongly when others did not view or treat him in a special way.

As an adult, Brad was able to use his narcissistic strategies at work. The employees of the small plumbing company he owned had to either tolerate his narcissistic behavior or to look for another job (as many did). His wife and child also bore the brunt of his constant bragging, unreasonable demands, and frequent put-downs. At age 65, Brad sold his company, retired, and began to spend much more time at home. His wife, who could not tolerate increased exposure to his obnoxious behaviors, separated from him, and his grown son, from whom he had grown increasingly alienated, wanted nothing to do with him. He soon found himself without meaningful work or relationships. His former "friends" were actually men whose wives socialized with his wife and him because they liked his wife. Once he and his wife separated, they no longer had to tolerate his boorish, egotistical, and critical behavior. Although Brad became somewhat depressed, he did not enter treatment for his dysphoria. He came only because his wife threatened divorce if he did not.

Brad was a challenging patient in treatment. His beliefs and emotions could fluctuate from moment to moment. Bragging about his financial success made him feel momentarily superior to the therapist. Perceiving that, as a patient, he was in a lower status position compared to the therapist, he felt quite inferior, which was intolerable to him. Thus he initially put his therapist down at every opportunity, became angry when she did not agree to his entitled requests, and resented being asked to do therapy homework.

SUMMARY

It is important for therapists to be aware of the typical beliefs and strategies associated with each personality disorder. This understanding prompts therapists to look for and categorize the multitude of data that patients present so they can conceptualize patients and plan treatment across sessions and instantly decide what to do, moment by moment, within sessions. An awareness of the beliefs and behavioral strategies of patients who have personality disorders is also often critical in establishing and maintaining a strong therapeutic alliance, as described in the next two chapters.

CHAPTER 4

Developing and Using the Therapeutic Alliance

Effective cognitive therapy requires a good therapeutic alliance. While a small number of patients may not care much about a therapist's "bedside manner" and just want tools to overcome their distress, many patients will not acquire or use new skills to change their cognitions, behavior, and emotional responses unless such learning takes place in the context of a supportive, empathic relationship. And the therapeutic relationship itself can be a vehicle for helping these patients develop a more positive view of themselves and others and learn that interpersonal problems can be solved.

This chapter covers many aspects of the therapeutic alliance. The first section describes patients' predictions about treatment to help explain why it is relatively easy to develop a good working relationship with some patients and why it is more difficult to do so with others. The second section presents essential strategies to use with all patients. The following section describes how to identify problems in the alliance, especially when patients do not directly reveal their discomfort, and, having identified a problem, how to conceptualize the problem and plan strategy. The last section of this chapter describes how to *use* the therapeutic relationship to bring about change in patients' beliefs and behavioral strategies. Many of the principles outlined throughout the chapter are illustrated in a final case example. Chapter 5 illustrates common difficulties in the therapeutic alliance through specific case examples.

PATIENTS' PREDICTIONS ABOUT TREATMENT

It is relatively easy to build an alliance with patients who enter treatment with *benign* predictions about what their experience will be like. When patients have predominantly positive attitudes about other people, they frequently hold optimistic views about their therapist and about treatment:

> - "My therapist is likely to be understanding, caring, and competent."
> - "I will be able to do what my therapist asks."
> - "My therapist will see me in a positive light."
> - "Therapy will make me feel better."

Some patients with challenging problems, however, have generally negative ideas about other people and enter treatment with a different set of predictions:

> - "My therapist will hurt me."
> - "My therapist will criticize me."
> - "I'll fail."
> - "Therapy will make me feel worse."

Therapists invariably need to spend much more time building trust with this latter group of patients. And despite therapists' reasonable behavior, some patients do believe that their therapist has hurt them, perceiving (correctly or incorrectly) that their therapist has rejected, controlled, or manipulated them; invalidated their feelings; evaluated them negatively; or expected too much of them. Patients may then react in a variety of ways. Some may become anxious and avoid revealing (or, at worst, avoid coming to therapy altogether). Others may become angry, critical, demeaning, or accusatory toward their therapist.

As with most problems in therapy, difficulties in the therapeutic alliance may have a practical basis (the therapist is interrupting too much or too abruptly), a psychological basis (the patient has interfering beliefs such as "If my therapist doesn't give me 100%, it means she doesn't care"), or both.

STRATEGIES TO BUILD THE THERAPEUTIC ALLIANCE

Following certain basic cognitive therapy principles helps the therapist to establish and maintain the therapeutic relationship with patients:

> - Actively collaborate with the patient.
> - Demonstrate empathy, caring, and understanding.
> - Adapt one's therapeutic style.
> - Alleviate distress.
> - Elicit feedback at the end of sessions.

As described below, therapists need to assess the degree to which they are successfully implementing these strategies. And sometimes they need to vary these standard principles for patients who present challenging problems.

Actively Collaborate with the Patient

Therapists act as a team with patients. As such, they generally assume the role of guide with a certain expertise. Therapists and patients jointly make decisions about therapy—for example, which problems to focus on during sessions and how frequently to meet (in the absence of practical restraints). Therapists provide rationales for their interventions. Therapists and patients also engage in collaborative empiricism, in which they jointly investigate the validity of patients' thinking.

Sometimes a problem arises in the collaboration because of therapist error. Therapists may be too directive, overbearing, or confrontational. This type of problem may be identified by asking a colleague to listen to a therapy tape. Many times, however, a lack of collaboration is related to patients' perceptions. Some patients with challenging problems do not collaborate easily. Meredith, for example, became irritated when her therapist tried to interrupt her and steer her toward problem solving. She perceived her therapist as being overcontrolling. Her therapist had to compromise with her and allow her to talk uninterruptedly for the first part of each therapy session, before Meredith was willing to focus on a particular problem. On the other hand, Joshua, a dependent patient, was overly passive in session, believing that his therapist should unilaterally make all decisions since he perceived himself as incapable of prioritizing problems for the agenda or responding to his dysfunctional thoughts. Joshua's therapist had to encourage him to take a more active role.

Demonstrate Empathy, Caring, Optimism, Genuineness, Accurate Understanding, and Competence

Effective cognitive therapy requires therapists to possess and use all these essential counseling skills. Review of a therapy tape can reveal whether a therapist is indeed demonstrating these qualities. It is important to note, however, that therapists often need to fine-tune the degree to which they directly display these qualities to patients. It is essential to be alert to the patient's affective experience from moment to moment in therapy to determine how best to proceed.

Most patients respond quite positively to direct expressions of empathy. They feel supported and understood, and the therapeutic alliance becomes stronger. Some, however, may actually feel worse, at least at times. Jenny, a depressed patient with histrionic features, sometimes cried in session, while she recounted one interpersonal problem after another. Whenever her therapist provided too much direct empathy, she just cried harder, as she misperceived her therapists' words as validating the hopelessness of her situation.

Likewise, most patients benefit from genuine expressions of caring, but some do not, particularly early in treatment. Lloyd, an autonomous patient with schizoid features, felt acutely uncomfortable when his therapist expressed her caring early in treatment. Danielle, a paranoid patient, became highly suspicious when her therapist made positive comments about her. Sandy, an avoidant patient, became distressed when her therapist expressed direct empathy to her in their first session because she feared her therapist would become angry with her when he discovered that Sandy was actually bad and unworthy of being cared about.

Patients generally respond positively when their therapist maintains a consistently upbeat attitude about the probability that therapy will help. Others, however, respond negatively, especially those who believe that such optimism is unwarranted and demonstrates their therapists' lack of understanding about them and their difficulties.

Most patients react positively when their therapists reinforce them for making changes in their thinking and behavior. When Julian's therapist praised him for getting out of bed and straightening up his apartment, though, he perceived her as being condescending. When Sandy's therapist gave her positive feedback, she became anxious, fearing that her therapist would now have increasingly greater expectations of her that she would be unable to fulfill.

Accurate understanding of the patients' experience and an ability to communicate this understanding are essential, as is the judgment about when and in how much detail to share this understanding with patients. Some patients become distressed if their therapists present inaccurate conceptualizations—or present accurate conceptualizations prematurely, before they have developed sufficient trust in the therapist. Craig became highly threatened when his couple therapist presented a hypothesis early in treatment. She suggested that perhaps he became so angry with his wife for minor infractions because her refusal to accommodate to him was an indication to him that he was weak. While this conceptualization later proved accurate, the therapist should not have presented it so early in treatment to this particular patient, who had a fragile sense of self. The therapist had failed to pick up Craig's verbal and nonverbal cues that indicated he was becoming increasingly uncomfortable in the session.

Most patients respond well when their therapist maintains a quiet air of competence and confidence. To others, though, this attitude is unsettling. When William's therapist remained unruffled by his overt skepticism, he perceived her as acting "superior" in order to make him feel small.

Adapt One's Therapeutic Style to Patients' Special Characteristics

Therapists need to vary their style for some patients. Ongoing supervision with review of therapy tapes may be required to identify this particular therapeutic problem. While many patients will likely respond well to a therapist's natural style, others—particularly those who present challenges in treatment—will not. For example, a patient with narcissistic personality disorder may respond better when a therapist is somewhat deferential. When Jerry initially showed off his expensive designer suit to the therapist, she unashamedly confessed her ignorance of the designer and asked him questions deliberately intended to allow him to feel superior to her. An avoidant patient generally builds trust in his therapist when she initially does not push him to reveal sensitive material. A dependent patient usually appreciates a therapist who takes charge in the session and is fairly directive, while a patient with obsessive–compulsive personality disorder generally does not. While most patients are comforted by the therapist's direct expressions of caring, paranoid patients may become suspicious and on guard.

Some patients respond well when the therapist makes therapeutic self-disclosures. Others wonder why the therapist is wasting their time. Reluctant patients sometimes feel more comfortable when their therapist initially takes a more academic approach to therapy. Some patients are comfortable getting right down to problem solving. Others need much more empathy and support along with problem solving. Therapists must be aware that part of the art of cognitive therapy is recognizing when patients are uncomfortable with their therapists' style (described later in this chapter) and then modifying their behavior accordingly.

Alleviate Distress

One of the best ways to strengthen the therapeutic alliance is to help patients solve their problems and improve their mood. In fact, DeRubeis and Feeley (1990) found that patients perceived their therapists as empathic *following* an improvement in their symptoms. A tenuous alliance may be strengthened considerably when patients recognize that they feel better by the end of a session and especially when they notice that they are functioning better during the week. Assessing patients' mood at the beginning and end of sessions and reviewing changes in functioning over the past week can indicate whether therapists are achieving this objective. One exception to this principle, however, is the patient who fears that if he gets better in therapy, his life will get worse (e.g., he is worried that he will have to start taking on responsibilities he does not want to assume or that he will have to face the likelihood that a highly unsatisfying marriage may never significantly improve).

Elicit Feedback

Some patients have dysfunctional reactions to therapists that interfere with their gaining full benefit from a therapy session. Therapists often need to elicit patients' thoughts when they notice negative affect shifts during the session and to spend considerable effort to uncover a therapeutic relationship problem and improve the alliance. These kinds of patients are described more fully in the next section.

It is sufficient, however, to ask many patients for feedback toward the end of therapy sessions. Patients who have not previously been treated with cognitive therapy are often amazed and pleased that their therapists are willing to open themselves up to criticism or correction and to modify their treatment. Eliciting patients' reactions can greatly improve the alliance—and provide valuable information the therapist can use to make therapy more effective.

It is important for therapists to ask patients for feedback in a *nonperfunctory* way, using questions such as:

- "What did you think about today's session?"
- "Was there anything you thought I got wrong or didn't understand?"
- "Is there anything you want to do differently next session?"

It is useful to have some patients fill out a feedback form immediately following therapy sessions (see J. Beck, 2005, for an example). The form directs the patient to reflect on the important content and process of therapy, and to evaluate the therapist on dimensions of caring and competence. Valuable information can be gleaned from the form, particularly if therapists stress how helpful it is to receive positive feedback when warranted and also *negative* feedback when the patient thinks the therapist could be more helpful. Some patients are willing to provide honest feedback in this written form that they were not willing to provide verbally.

Therapists may also elicit feedback toward the beginning of sessions *if they suspect or know that the patient had a negative reaction to the previous session.* Ken, for example, had seemed somewhat irritable in the previous session but had denied it. At the next session, his therapist asked, "I was thinking over last session and I realized that I had been pushing you pretty hard about considering getting a different job. Did it feel like that to you, too?"

When patients are still reluctant to provide feedback, it may be important to identify their dysfunctional beliefs about revealing, as described in the next section.

IDENTIFYING AND SOLVING PROBLEMS
IN THE THERAPEUTIC ALLIANCE

In order to solve difficulties in the therapeutic relationship, therapists need to identify the existence of a problem, conceptualize why it arose, and, based on this understanding and a general conceptualization of the patient, plan a strategy to correct it, as described below.

Identifying a Therapeutic Alliance Problem

Sometimes problems in the therapeutic relationship are obvious. One patient loudly questions his therapist's motives or expertise. Another blatantly lies to the therapist (see Newman & Strauss, 2003, for more on this specific problem). A third patient accuses the therapist of not caring about her. But signs of a possible therapeutic relationship problem are often more subtle, and the therapist may not know whether there is a problem—and if so, whether it is related to the alliance. Patients may avert their gaze and hesitate before speaking. They may suddenly look more distressed. Their body language may indicate that they are trying to protect themselves.

Therefore, it is essential to be attuned to patients' emotional states and to their shifts of affect during the therapy session. Negative changes in the patients' body language, facial expression, tone of voice, and choice of words can indicate that patients have just had automatic thoughts that could potentially interfere with treatment. When therapists note these changes, they can use standard questions to elicit patients' emotions and automatic thoughts:

> ■ "How are you feeling right now?"
> ■ "What just went through your mind?"

Patients who have the following kinds of automatic thoughts are unlikely to gain sufficient benefit from the session:

> - "My therapist doesn't understand me."
> - "My therapist doesn't care about me."
> - "My therapist isn't listening to me."
> - "My therapist is trying to control me."
> - "My therapist is judging me."
> - "My therapist should 'fix' me."

Robin, for example, started to look nervous during a therapy session. She began to bounce her leg and her face looked drawn. Through questioning, her therapist discovered she was thinking, "If I tell my therapist about [my sexual history], she'll judge me. She probably won't like me. She may not want to see me any more."

It is important to note that many affect shifts are *not* related to an alliance problem. Patients may express automatic thoughts about themselves ("I'm a mess"), about treatment ("This is too hard"), or about their difficulties ("What if I can't solve my problems?").

Likewise, patients may display behavior that interferes with treatment. It is important to note, though, that problematic behavior may or may not be related to a problem in the therapeutic alliance. One patient failed to do his homework, for example, because he predicted he would not do it well and that his therapist would criticize him. Another patient, though, had a solid alliance with his therapist but was too disorganized at home to do his assignment. Again, it is important to ask patients what they were thinking just before they engaged in the dysfunctional behavior—or just before they failed to engage in a functional behavior.

If therapists suspect that there is an alliance problem the patient has not acknowledged, they can normalize the problem and probe further:

> ■ "Some patients don't like the idea of doing homework because they feel like I'm telling them what to do. Could something like that be going on with you, too?"

The examples below illustrate how the therapist determined whether patients' behavior indicated a problem with the alliance.

Example 1: Patient Continually Says "I Don't Know"

Tom, a 15-year-old depressed adolescent, often said, "I don't know" in the first session. Toward the beginning of the second session, he again answered, "I don't know" when his therapist asked him whether anything had changed at school.

THERAPIST: Did that question [I just asked] make you uncomfortable?

TOM: (*Shrugs.*)

THERAPIST: I'm wondering whether you truly *don't* know—or if there's something *good* about saying "I don't know." (*pause*) For example, then maybe I will stop bothering you with annoying questions?

TOM: (*Smiles.*)

THERAPIST: You're smiling. Am I right? Do you wish I'd stop pestering you? Would you rather not be here?

TOM: Yeah, I guess.

Here the therapist confirms her suspicion that the patient does not feel a positive connection to her and indeed would rather not be in treatment. Another patient answered the same question in a different way: "No, it's not that your questions are annoying. I'm just so confused these days." In the absence of any other data indicating a problem in the therapeutic alliance, the therapist conceptualized that the problem needed a practical solution. She solved the problem by making her questions more specific.

Example 2: Patient Does Not Answer Questions in a Straightforward Manner

Jodi's therapist noticed that Jodi frequently failed to answer questions directly when she felt uncomfortable. When Jodi displayed the same kind of behavior for the third time, the therapist addressed the problem directly:

THERAPIST: (*summarizing*) So maybe there *is* reason to believe that you can influence your husband more than you first thought?

JODI: You see, he's always been like this. I should have paid more attention when we were dating. I mean, he was doing the same stuff then.

THERAPIST: (*drawing her back*) What do you think of the idea that you can influence him now?

JODI: He's like that with his mother, too.

THERAPIST: Jodi, how did you feel when I suggested that you have might have some influence? (*pause*) Did you feel a little anxious?

JODI: (*Thinks; sighs.*) I don't know.

THERAPIST: What did it mean to you when I said it?

JODI: I don't know.

THERAPIST: I take it, it wasn't good, though.

JODI: No. (*Thinks.*) See, I guess I still don't really know if I should stay with him or leave.

In this case, the therapist conceptualized that the patient did not answer his questions directly because Jodi was ambivalent about her marriage. While there was not a rupture in the therapeutic alliance, Jodi clearly did not want her therapist to explore the possibility that she might be able to make the relationship with her husband better.

Example 3: Patient Changes the Subject

In another case, the therapist ascertained that a patient's failure to answer some questions directly was not related to a therapeutic alliance problem, but rather to the patient's verbal style:

THERAPIST: I felt like I was interrupting you a lot today. Did that bother you?

PATIENT: No, it was okay.

THERAPIST: I was trying to figure out when you changed the subject a few times whether you didn't want to keep talking about, say, the problem with your sister.

PATIENT: I did want to talk about that. I guess I was just going off on a tangent again. My wife says I do that a lot.

Conceptualizing the Problem and Planning Strategy

In order to make therapeutic decisions about how best to strengthen the therapeutic alliance, therapists should assess how serious the problem is and whether it is better to ignore the problem, to address it immediately, or to address it later. In order to formulate a strategy, therapists must conceptualize why the problem arose. As mentioned previously, some problems arise due to therapist error, some arise because of patients' beliefs, and some are a combination of the two.

Determining the Extent and Immediacy of the Problem

When therapists decide that a problem is related to the therapeutic alliance, they must next decide how much time and effort should be spent on it. A good rule of thumb is to make the relationship *strong enough* for patients to be willing to collaborate with the therapist and work toward their goals. *Spending more time on the therapeutic relationship than is needed means spending less time helping patients solve their real-life problems.* (On the other hand, as described at the end of this chapter, a positive therapeutic relationship can be a powerful tool in modifying patients' dysfunctional beliefs about themselves and others—and there may be a strong rationale for focusing more attention on it.)

It is sometimes quite apparent that a therapeutic alliance problem is acute and needs to be immediately addressed—for example in the case of a patient who expresses anger toward the therapist, a patient who is so anxious that she can barely speak, or a patient who dominates the session so much that the therapist can not get a word in edgewise. Often these kinds of problems require significant attention and remediation. Harold, for example, was upset with his therapist for jumping in to solve his problems. The therapist needed to do several things to repair the relationship: she had to take care to be more overtly empathic toward him, she had to negotiate the structure of the session (offering him an opportunity to talk uninterruptedly for a period of time), and she had to modify Harold's perception that she didn't really care about him as a person and only wanted to work in a business-like way to "fix" him.

Some problems in the alliance, however, occur infrequently or are relatively minor. Many of these kinds of problems can be resolved in the course of the session. Martin became legitimately annoyed when his therapist forgot a significant issue from the previous session. A simple apology—"I'm sorry, I should have remembered that"—solved the problem. Holly looked quite distressed at her second therapy session when her therapist suggested several homework assignments; she predicted that she would fail to do them well and that she would let the therapist down. Her therapist was able to solve the problem quickly, by suggesting that two of the assignments be optional. He wisely did not intervene further at this point, concluding that if her reaction later proved to be typical and problematic, he could address it at that time.

Still other problems can be ignored, at least for the moment. George, an adolescent boy, rolled his eyes when his therapist suggested that perhaps he clarify an assignment with his teacher. She ignored this mildly negative reaction and went on to question him about classmates who might be able to help him figure out what to do, which the patient found more palatable.

When therapists see dysfunctional *patterns* in the therapeutic alliance, more work on the relationship is often required. Michael (a transcript for whom appears at the end of this chapter) became mildly annoyed with his therapist when she positively reinforced him and gave him some basic information about depression. After the first and second incident, she apologized and moved on. When he displayed a negative reaction for the third time, she delved into the meaning to him of what she had just said, elicited a dysfunctional belief, and modified it in the context of their relationship (and several other relationships he had as well).

Conceptualizing Why the Problem Arose

Having conceptualized that it is important to address a problem in the therapeutic alliance, therapists next need to determine whether the problem arose because they themselves made an error or because patients' dysfunctional beliefs became activated, or both.

When the Therapist Has Made an Error

It is important for therapists to recognize that difficulties in the therapeutic relationship may be related to their own behaviors or attitudes. While asking patients for honest feedback may provide this necessary information, at times it is essential for therapists to ask colleagues to review a tape of the therapy session to determine the extent to which the therapist is the cause of a problem.

When therapists realize that they have made a mistake, it is usually appropriate and helpful for them to say they are sorry. Nondefensive apologizing is an important skill to model for many patients with challenging problems. For example, Bob became distressed when his therapist interrupted him several times in a short period of time. When he told her that she was not letting him relate what he believed he needed to, his therapist apologized. Bob indeed was correct; his therapist had misjudged Bob's need to unburden himself. Her apology served to strengthen their alliance.

Keith had been anxious because he had not been able to carry out a therapy homework assignment. His therapist realized that she had been in error; she had suggested an assignment that was too difficult for him. When she acknowledged and apologized for her error, his anxiety lessened and his trust in her grew.

When Patients' Dysfunctional Beliefs Interfere with the Alliance

Difficulties in the therapeutic alliance may also be related to patients' general dysfunctional beliefs about themselves, others, and relationships, and to the strategies they employ to cope with these beliefs. Some patients may believe, for example, that their therapist is likely to be critical of them. If this belief is specific to the therapist, and not to people in general, the belief may be easily changed. If, on the other hand, the belief is a subset of a broader belief about people in general ("Other people are highly likely to be critical"), it may interfere with using standard cognitive therapy.

Therapists first need to identify patients' interfering beliefs and plan a strategy, based on a sound conceptualization. Directly eliciting and testing beliefs may be indicated for some patients. Covertly identifying and working around the beliefs (e.g., modifying treatment to avoid activating the belief) may be more helpful for other patients. In either case, therapists usually need to use a number of interventions over time, as illustrated in the following case examples.

Case Example 1

Brent, a 35-year-old depressed patient with narcissistic personality disorder, believed that he was basically inferior and that others were superior, though he covered up these beliefs of inferiority with demonstrations of his superiority and entitled demands. He continually believed that others would disrespect him. Small events, even neutral ones, often sent him into a rage: a clerk failed to thank him for payment; an usher pointed out his seat rather than showing him to it; a man in an elevator did not hold the "Open Door" button for him; the manager of a store asked him to leave at closing time.

The same beliefs that became activated in his dealings with others also became activated during treatment itself. Because he was coming to therapy for help, he automatically felt in an inferior position. He assumed his therapist would see herself as superior and him as inferior—and treat him as an inferior. He was hypervigilant for putdowns and misread his therapist's intentions. He tried to belittle her, making "jokes" about the furniture in her office, asking her if she knew the meaning of arcane psychological terms, acting surprised when she had not heard of his favorite classical music artist, stating that his previous therapists were more skilled than she was. He also acted inappropriately sullen when his therapist did not accede to his requests for special favors such as setting appointments outside of the therapist's usual hours. Brent tried to impress his therapist with his superiority in various ways: using sophisticated vocabulary, pointing out his high-status clothing, bragging about minor accomplishments at work.

His therapist conceptualized that if she confronted him about his critical remarks early in treatment, she would probably further activate his beliefs of inferiority. Instead she took pains to react nondefensively. When Brent asserted that she was less skilled than his previous therapists, she asked, "Can you tell me what they did that I don't do so I can help you more?" When he asked her about a psychological concept with which she was unfamiliar, she said, "I don't know about that. I probably should, though. What *does* it refer to?" When he made jokes about the appearance of her office, she laughed with him and made a joke herself: "You know, I knew I should have gotten an MBA. Then I could have had great furniture!"

In this way, the therapist accomplished several therapeutic goals. She directly modeled nondefensive behavior and demonstrated that it is possible to take criticism and put-downs without a diminishment in one's self-esteem. Failing to criticize or put Brent down decreased his sense of vulnerability and increased his sense of trust in the therapist, thereby strengthening the therapeutic alliance. Over time, after many different kinds of interventions, Brent began to change his beliefs. He felt less and less of a need to use his dysfunctional coping strategies with his therapist. He also began to believe that perhaps not everyone would put him down. He became more willing to try behavioral experiments outside of therapy in which he did not try to diminish other people before they had, in his mind, the opportunity to diminish him first.

Brent's therapist had conceptualized that she needed to work around Brent's beliefs initially. The mere act of identifying these cognitions would have activated them too strongly. Later in therapy, his therapist was able to elicit and modify his beliefs more directly, using standard belief modification strategies (see Chapter 13).

Case Example 2

Claire was a 42-year-old patient with major depression superimposed on lifelong dysthymia and passive-aggressive features. She saw herself as weak, somewhat ineffectual, and lazy, while she viewed others as strong, intrusive, and demanding. She generally tried to exert control by displaying irritability when she was asked to do something she did not want to do or by outwardly assenting to others' requests, but then either fulfilling the request insufficiently, or poorly, or not at all. Often when her husband asked her to do chores she disliked, such as balancing the checkbook or running errands, he ended up having to do them himself. Hypersensitive to control, she found ways to undermine her husband's authority when he set reasonable limits with their child.

Claire found it relatively easy to secure part-time jobs but had a history of lasting only a few months before she was fired for failing to live up to her bosses' expectations. She had strained relationships with her family of origin; unlike her siblings, she would either not show up at family events or come very late; she refused to contribute to the physical care of her aging parents.

Claire's dysfunctional beliefs about control became activated during therapy sessions. She perceived that she was weak and her therapist was trying to control her. She spent considerable time in session complaining about her husband, her bosses, and other people. She resisted taking a problem-solving approach. Although she and her therapist collaboratively set homework assignments, Claire invariably did not do them, saying she had lost her therapy notes, her week had been too busy, or she had come to realize that the homework would not really help.

Claire's therapist quickly conceptualized that Claire was using coping strategies to avoid the activation of distressing beliefs. She confirmed her hypothesis directly: "Claire, sometimes when I make suggestions to people about things they could do at home, they feel like I'm trying to control them. (*pause*) Do you ever feel like that?" When Claire acknowledged that she did, the therapist responded empathically, "That must feel bad. We should try something different, then. Do you have any ideas?" When Claire shook her head, her therapist said, "You know, I wonder whether it might be helpful to go over your goals for therapy again and make sure you really want to accomplish them. If you do, we can try to figure out how you can do that in a way that doesn't feel so controlling to you. (*pause*) Is that okay?"

When they reviewed the goal list, the therapist asked Claire to rank the goals in order of importance. Claire related that she most wanted to engage in more pleasurable activities such as seeing friends, reading, and exploring topics of interest on the Internet. She had almost stopped doing these as her depression deepened. Her therapist then gave her a choice of discussing in session what she could do this week or figuring it out on her own at home. Claire chose the latter and indeed reported at the next session that she had done several activities.

Progress in therapy soon slowed as Claire began to feel better. Her therapist helped her identify and respond to an interfering belief: "If I feel better, my therapist and husband will have greater and greater expectations of me." Evaluation of this belief, simple problem solving, and role playing reassured Claire that she would be able to assert herself if such a problem arose, and she was able to make further progress.

One essential lesson for many patients with challenging problems to learn is that interpersonal problems can be improved or resolved through adopting a more accurate, functional perspective on others' behavior and/or through direct problem solving, for example, by changing one's behavior toward others or by asking others to modify their behavior.

USING THE THERAPEUTIC RELATIONSHIP TO ACHIEVE THERAPEUTIC GOALS

There are many strategies therapists can use to strengthen the therapeutic alliance and simultaneously achieve other therapeutic goals. In this section, strategies in three important areas are described: providing positive relationship experiences, working through alliance problems, and generalizing what the patient has learned from working through problems in the therapeutic relationship to other important relationships in the patient's life.

Providing Positive Relationship Experiences

Patients with challenging problems may have disturbed relationships, accompanied by dysfunctional beliefs about themselves and others. The therapy session provides a number of opportunities for therapists to correct patients' negative beliefs. Therapists can help patients reinforce a more positive (actually a more realistic) view of themselves and others in many ways, including:

- Using positive reinforcement.
- Using self-disclosure.
- Reducing the inequality in the therapeutic relationship.
- Disagreeing with the patient's negative self-view.
- Providing realistic hope.
- Directly expressing empathy and caring.
- Expressing regret about therapeutic limitations.
- Helping patients recognize the therapist's sense of connectedness.

Therapists can also help patients change their view of others by demonstrating that they will not hurt them and by modeling good interpersonal problem solving (Safran & Muran, 2000).

Using Positive Reinforcement

It is important for therapists not only to directly express empathy and support, but also to provide positive reinforcement when patients make adaptive changes in their thinking, mood, or behavior or when they display attitudes or behaviors that indicate their positive qualities. As standard practice, cognitive therapists ask patients toward the beginning of therapy sessions to tell them (in addition to what difficulties they encountered) the positive things they had done or the positive things that had happened to them since the previous session. They also ask patients to relate what they had been able to do for homework. Such a review provides opportunities for therapists to reinforce the patient.

- "I'm glad you . . . [went to that party and had a good time]."
- "I hope you're proud that you were able to . . . [make it through your exams]."
- "How wonderful that you . . . [helped your neighbor when she needed you]."
- "It's impressive that you . . . [could answer back your negative thoughts when he said that and feel better]."
- "That's such a wonderful quality you have, being able to . . . [comfort people as you do]."
- "Not everyone can . . . [handle that kind of criticism as well as you]."
- "That's good that you . . . [made yourself get out of bed almost every day this week]."
- "Did you give yourself credit for . . . [doing these things instead of hurting yourself]?"
- "If only everyone could . . . [figure out what their children really need, as you can]."

Encouraging statements such as these can undermine patients' beliefs of helplessness, unlovability, and unworthiness. They can also reinforce patients' beliefs that their therapist is supportive and caring.

Using Self-Disclosure

Judicious use of self-disclosure can help strengthen the therapeutic alliance and provide an important vehicle for learning. Claudia was quite upset because her husband was about to take a job with a much higher level of responsibility, which meant that he would not be home for dinner many nights with her and their children. Her therapist related how she had dealt with the same problem several years earlier: by thinking of her husband's job as shift work, meaning that he was expected to work late hours and did not have a choice if he wanted to keep his job. Claudia appreciated the willingness of her therapist to share this personal information and felt a stronger bond with her.

The therapist's disclosure also indirectly helped Claudia recognize that she was not the only one who had had to face such a situation and that Claudia had a choice of whether to continue to agonize about the problem or to think about it in another way and feel better. Claudia was able to adopt the same viewpoint toward her husband's hours, and indeed her distress diminished. She was then able to engage in productive problem solving with her therapist to figure out ways to manage her children more effectively in the early evening.

In another case, Eileen, an autonomous patient who was significantly depressed, was feeling overwhelmed at the thought of having to replace some furniture that had been damaged in a flood. Her therapist normalized the problem by relating that she, like several other people she knew, had had a similar problem. The therapist explained that she had finally solved the problem by asking a friend to help her and also by realizing that she needed to buy furniture that was acceptable but not necessarily perfect. Eileen felt heartened to discover that her difficulty was common and she began to believe that if it was all right for her therapist to ask for help, maybe it was all right for her, too.

Redressing the Balance in the Therapeutic Relationship

It is important to help patients who feel particularly one down to redress the imbalance in the therapeutic relationship. Gil, who generally believed that he was a failure compared to others, felt more competent and less inferior when his therapist asked him questions about his job as a customer service representative and noted his patience and ability to work with a difficult supervisor and irate customers. Keith's therapist told him how impressed she was that he knew so much about opera and classical music. Laura, a chronically depressed patient, had much difficulty functioning from day to day, and sometimes could not take care of her home. She usually felt better when her therapist deliberately asked questions about her dogs. A new dog owner herself, Laura's therapist knew little about caring for and training dogs, an area in which Laura excelled. Soliciting Laura's advice and telling her how well her suggestions had worked helped Laura to feel more competent.

Disagreeing with Patients' Negative Beliefs

It is important for a therapist to acknowledge that patients' beliefs make sense given their experience—but that the therapist, a more objective observer, does not necessarily agree with them. When June expressed hopelessness that she could ever feel better, her therapist reassured her that she did not hold the same view:

THERAPIST: Oh, *now* I understand why you would be so hopeless about ever feeling better. I'm sure if those things had happened to me and I believed those things about myself, I'd be pretty hopeless, too. But while *you* may believe that you're bad because of how your dad treated you, I want you to know that *I* don't believe you're bad, not for a *minute*. It was obviously *he* who was troubled—*not you*! (*long pause*) What do you think about that?

Providing Understanding Combined with Realistic Optimism

Patients who have experienced emotional deprivation often need significant nurturance, empathy, and support from their therapists. It is important to recognize that empathy alone can sometimes lead to patients' feeling worse if they perceive, correctly or not, that the therapist believes they have been unalterably affected by adverse (and sometimes devastating) life events. To forestall such a perception, the therapist may need to couple empathic statements with other statements that express at least guarded optimism for the future.

- "I'm so sorry that happened to you. *No one*, least of all *you*, deserves something like that. (*gently*) But I *am* glad you came to see me so I can help you with this."
- "That must have been so difficult—and I know you're still in a lot of pain because of it. (*pause*) Now you might not be hopeful, but I have to let you know that *I* am hopeful we can decrease the pain."
- "No *wonder* that's so difficult for you. . . . It's now becoming clear to me that we have to break this [task] down, go slower, make it easier . . . . How does that sound?"

Of course, it is important to watch for patients' reactions to such statements. Some may be suspicious of or discount what the therapist is saying or even feel that the therapist is trivializing their problems. Patients with these perceptions generally show a change of affect, providing the alert therapist with an opportunity to elicit their thoughts and associated meanings and respond to them effectively.

CASE EXAMPLE

Meredith, a patient with chronic depression and post-traumatic stress disorder, had been physically and sexually abused as a child by her father. Her mother aided and abetted in the abuse. Meredith developed very strong beliefs that she was bad, unlovable, and unworthy. Her therapist used many strategies over time to help her modify these beliefs, including many therapeutic relationship interventions. For example, her therapist made considerable effort to engage Meredith conversationally about her volunteer work at church, about her (very positive) relationship with her child, about her interest in the plight of refugees. These conversations gave the therapist the opportunity to show her interest in and respect for Meredith and to positively reinforce the patient for her compassionate traits. The therapist was also able to use data gleaned from these conversations later in treatment as evidence that Meredith's new core belief, that she was an okay person, was valid.

Expressing Regret about Therapeutic Limitations

It is sometimes helpful for therapists to state that they are sorry that they can not do more for the patient: "I wish I had the power to take away your pain" or "I'm sorry I can't be your therapist *and* your friend." Then it is important to follow it up with a more positive statement: "I would like to see what we can do, though, to *reduce* your pain." "If I had to be one versus the other, though, I'm glad to be your therapist so I can keep working hard to help you."

Helping Patients Recognize Therapists' Sense of Connectedness

Therapists sometimes need to express their continuing state of connectedness to the patient, directly and indirectly. For example, they may indicate to patients that they are not forgotten between sessions.

> ◼ "I was thinking about you this week. And it occurred to me that it might help if we _____ this session."

This kind of statement sends a message that the therapist cares, does not forget the patient when her appointment is over, is motivated to think about her when she is not in the office, and is dedicated to helping her more than she may know.

Patients often feel less connected to people in general when they are depressed. They may feel less connected to their therapists as well. Therapists need to be alert to this possibility, particularly when working with patients whose depression increases significantly during treatment. Often patients recognize that they feel less connected and they assume that their therapists are also feeling less connected. Therapists can usually uncover this problem through direct questioning:

THERAPIST: You seem a little different this week. I wonder, are you feeling less connected to therapy and to me?

PATIENT: Yeah, I guess so.

THERAPIST: Are you also thinking that *I* feel less connected to *you?*

PATIENT: (*Thinks.*) Yeah.

THERAPIST: I'm so glad you told me that. So let me tell you the truth. If anything, I feel *more* connected to you now. I feel badly that you're more depressed—and I want to help you even more. (*pause*) Okay?

PATIENT: Okay.

WORKING THROUGH THERAPEUTIC ALLIANCE PROBLEMS AND GENERALIZING TO OTHER RELATIONSHIPS

When difficulties in the therapeutic relationship are related to patients' dysfunctional beliefs, therapists have the opportunity to gain insight about the distorted way in which patients see the therapist—and, quite possibly, other people. Eliciting and evaluating the validity of their beliefs about the therapist can strengthen the therapeutic alliance. The therapist often also has the opportunity to model good interpersonal problem solving. Many patients have not learned this skill; many have never really had the experience of solving relationship problems in a reasonable way. Indeed, one of the most important lessons for patients with a history of interpersonal difficulties is that when people are of good will, they can solve interpersonal problems. Generalizing what they have learned to other people helps patients develop more functional relationships outside of therapy.

The first part of this section describes a format that can be used when patients become distressed with therapists. The second part describes how therapists can use the therapeutic relationship to give constructive feedback to patients about their interpersonal behavior.

When Patients Are Distressed with the Therapist

When a significant problem has developed in the therapeutic relationship, the following may be a useful format to follow. The example provided is from a therapy session with a patient who has become angry at her therapist for trying to limit the patient's noncrisis phone calls between sessions.

- Elicit, then summarize, the patient's distorted automatic thoughts in the context of the cognitive model ("So when I brought up the topic of phone calls, you had the thought, '[My therapist] doesn't care,' and you felt hurt and angry. Is that right? How much did you believe that thought when you had it? How much do you believe it now?").

- Help the patient test the validity of automatic thoughts and alternative viewpoints through Socratic questioning ("What is the evidence that I don't care? Is there evidence on the other side? Is there an alternative explanation for what has happened here?").

- Encourage the patient to question the therapist directly ("It's *so* important for you to find out whether this idea that I don't care is true or not. How could you find out? How about asking me directly?").

- Provide direct, genuinely positive feedback ("Of *course* I care about you. The reason that I need to limit phone calls between sessions is that I need to keep a balanced life so *I* can be balanced and able to help you and my other patients enough.").

- Do problem solving ("How about if we figure out what else you *can* do when you get really upset? I don't want you to just wait for the next session and keep suffering.").

- Identify/modify dysfunctional assumptions ("So, to summarize, it sounds as if you had a really upsetting idea, 'If [my therapist] *really* cared, she'd help me whenever I'm upset, regardless of what she's doing.' What's another way of looking at this?").

- Evaluate assumptions in the context of other relationships ("Do you ever have this idea about other people? That if *they* really cared, they would do whatever it takes when you're upset? Does this idea ever make you upset with them, too? Whom *do* you have this idea about? Do you see it any differently now?").

- Have the patient summarize her new learning and write it down to review at home.

When Patients Need Feedback about Their Interpersonal Style

It is useful for therapists to use their own negative reactions to patients as a cue to assess the degree to which patients' behavior and attitudes in the session are representative of their behavior and attitudes outside of the session. Therapists can often gain insight into patients' difficulties and the way in which people in their environment likely react to them. If a therapist develops a strong reaction to the patient in their limited time together, it is likely that others, especially those who spend considerably more time with the patient, have reactions that are far greater (Newman & Ratto, 2003).

An important use of the therapeutic relationship can be for therapists to teach patients important interpersonal skills, for example, how to change their communication style when they are distressed (Layden, Newman, Freeman, & Morse, 1993). After several months of therapy Carrie, a patient with borderline personality disorder, had developed a reasonable therapeutic alliance with her therapist. At one particular session, though, Carrie became quite upset with her therapist when he asked her what ideas she had about solving a problem with Henry, a coworker. The therapist then offered several suggestions. Carrie calmed down and engaged in discussing her options. Afterwards, the therapist gave Carrie feedback about how she had initially expressed her distress—because he knew Carrie had a pattern of blaming others when she was dysphoric, which resulted in their withdrawal from her.

THERAPIST: Okay, feel good about the plan to deal with Henry?

CARRIE: Yeah.

THERAPIST: Is it all right if we go back for a minute? Do you remember what happened when you told me about the problem and I asked you if you had any ideas about how to solve it?

CARRIE: Yeah.

THERAPIST: What was going through your mind?

CARRIE: I guess I thought you expected me to figure out what to do—but I couldn't! That's why I brought it up in the first place!

THERAPIST: Oh, no wonder you were so upset. Was it the same kind of feeling you get sometimes with Peter [her husband]? Or with your mother?

CARRIE: Probably.

THERAPIST: Then I have some ideas about how you might be able to get their help better.

CARRIE: Okay.

THERAPIST: When you're really upset, you could say, as you did today, "You're not helping me enough! You don't understand!" Or you could say, "I'm feeling really overwhelmed. I really need your help." (*pause*) Do you see the difference? In the first one, the other person might get really defensive. In the second one, they might be much more motivated to help you." (*pause*) What do you think?

CARRIE: (*slowly*) I guess so.

THERAPIST: Do you want to think more about it this week?

CARRIE: Yeah.

SUMMARY CASE EXAMPLE

This final case example exemplifies many of the principles described in this section: apologizing to the patient, initially working around the activation of the patient's dysfunctional belief, identifying a pattern in his reactions to his therapist, modifying a dysfunctional belief about the therapist, and generalizing what the patient learned to others.

Michael's therapist engaged him in an extended discussion of a therapeutic relationship issue only *after* several instances in which he became annoyed with her during therapy when she positively reinforced him. In their third therapy session, Michael, a depressed patient, evinces displeasure with the therapist for the first time. Michael has just described the outcome of a behavioral experiment he had conducted for homework: being assertive to a coworker who was annoying him with her chatter.

MICHAEL: She seemed surprised and then she was a little distant for a couple of days but she's being less annoying now.

THERAPIST: So this idea that if you said something it would be too uncomfortable around her ... ?

MICHAEL: It wasn't great at first but it's okay now.

THERAPIST: I think what you did was really important. You had this negative assumption, you tested it out, and you found it wasn't true. And now you've made things better for yourself at work .... That's really good.

MICHAEL: (*Looks disgruntled.*)

THERAPIST: What just went through your mind when I said that?

MICHAEL: (*Takes a breath.*) That you're patronizing me.

THERAPIST: (*modeling apologizing*) Oh, I'm sorry if I came across that way. I didn't mean to. (*pause*) Is there anything else about work we should talk about?

MICHAEL: No, not really. (*Sighs.*) I just wish she'd quit.

THERAPIST: (*empathically*) Yeah, that might solve a lot of problems. (*pause*) Should we talk about your problem with getting organized at home now?

MICHAEL: Yeah, okay.

In the excerpt above, the therapist chose not to dwell on the patient's reaction to her. She merely apologized and went on. She and the patient were able to reestablish collaboration on another important problem. In the next session, the therapist reviewed the patient's (failed) attempts to engage in the exercise program they had discussed during the previous session. The patient again perceived that the therapist was patronizing him. The therapist indirectly assumed responsibility for the problem and refocused the patient.

MICHAEL: (*Sighs.*) I don't know what's wrong with me. I *know* I need to exercise. I'm getting all soft and flabby. I *know* I feel better when I do. I don't know how to get myself motivated.

THERAPIST: (*normalizing his experience and providing psychoeducation*) You know, a lot of people think they need to feel motivated *first*, *then* they can get themselves to do things. Actually it's the other way around. Most people just need to start *doing* it; then they feel more motivated.

MICHAEL: (*irritably*) I know, I know. You're not telling me anything new.

THERAPIST: (*acknowledging the patient's negative reaction*) Not so helpful, huh?

MICHAEL: No.

THERAPIST: (*hoping to reestablish collaboration by focusing on the problem in a different, more acceptable way*) Well, maybe it would be more helpful if we figured out what you were thinking this week that got in the way. When was a particular time this week that you even considered going to the gym?

The therapist next helps the patient identify his sabotaging thoughts and develop a robust response that he writes on an index card to read every day at home. Later in the session, the patient once again feels disgruntled.

MICHAEL: So I reminded myself that maybe it wasn't completely my fault that things weren't going so good with Julia [ex-girlfriend].

THERAPIST: And when you were able to tell yourself that, how did you feel?

MICHAEL: A little better. I mean, she isn't Miss Perfect either.

THERAPIST: That's really good. You were really able to affect your mood.

MICHAEL: (*Looks sour.*)

THERAPIST: Uh, oh. What just went through your mind?

MICHAEL: It just sounds so patronizing when you say things like that.

THERAPIST: Like . . . ?

MICHAEL: It's like you're patting me on the head. (*mimicking in an unpleasant tone*) "Good boy."

THERAPIST: Well, I'm glad that you told me . . . . Did I sound insincere? Is that it?

MICHAEL: No, it's more like you're complimenting me for doing such little things. It seems almost insulting. (*pause*) Not that I think you really *meant* to insult me.

THERAPIST: That's true. I didn't mean to. But what if it *were* true, that I *was* complimenting you for doing little things, what would be so bad about that?

MICHAEL: (*Looks down.*) I don't know.

THERAPIST: (*hypothesizing*) Does it make you feel kind of small, somehow? Like I'm the expert or bigger person being nice to someone smaller?

MICHAEL: (*Thinks.*) Yeah, something like that.

THERAPIST: Are you just saying that? Or do you really agree?

MICHAEL: No, I think that's right. It's like you're the teacher or something and I'm just the student.

THERAPIST: Well, I can see how that would be hard, then. And in a sense, you're right. I do have things to teach you . . . . On the other hand, I'd rather see us as a team.

MICHAEL: Hmm.

THERAPIST: So as a team, we have a problem to solve together. I guess I could stop saying positive things . . . but we'd have to figure out how you can know when you're on the right track. Or is there some other way you could see it when I do say positive things?

MICHAEL: Like what?

THERAPIST: I don't know . . . maybe that we're both doing well as a team?

MICHAEL: (*Thinks.*) No . . . I don't think that would do it.

THERAPIST: Well, this is a hard one. Could you think about it this week? Think about how you could feel better about my acknowledging what you do?

MICHAEL: Okay.

In this excerpt, the therapist senses that continuing to focus on the problem right then might not be productive, so she asks the patient to reflect on it between sessions. In the next session, the therapist assesses the degree to which it might be useful to delve into the beliefs underlying the problem in the therapeutic alliance.

THERAPIST: (*collaboratively*) I've been thinking some more about the problem we had last session when you felt I was patronizing you—is it okay if we talk about it a little more now?

MICHAEL: Okay.

THERAPIST: Were you able to come up with another way of looking at it?

MICHAEL: No, not really.

THERAPIST: Can I ask you this: This sense of being patronized, does it come up from time to time with other people? Or just with me?

MICHAEL: (*Thinks for several moments.*) No, not just with you. Ummm, I guess I feel it a lot with my boss. He's always explaining things way too much. He must think I'm stupid sometimes. (*pause*)

THERAPIST: And with anyone else?

MICHAEL: My parents, of course. I already told you, they always think they know better than I do. They're always telling me what to do.

THERAPIST: How about with Sharon [his girlfriend]? Ever feel patronized by her?

MICHAEL: (*Thinks.*) Not so much . . . wait . . . yeah, sometimes.

THERAPIST: For example?

MICHAEL: Like she'll have her opinion, say, of what movie we should go to, because she reads the entertainment section [of the newspaper]. And I'll say that I want to go to another movie that *I* heard was good and she'll say she knows it won't be very good because she read a review. One review—that's just one person's opinion and she believes it and so she doesn't want to go to the movie I want to go to.

THERAPIST: Well, that can be annoying. So I take it that if this sense of being small and patronized comes up from time to time.

MICHAEL: Yeah, I guess so.

THERAPIST: (*anticipating and heading off his response*) Do you think it's likely that you'll be able to make a major change in your boss, your parents, and Sharon?

MICHAEL: Maybe with Sharon, a little.

THERAPIST: And maybe with me, a little?

MICHAEL: Maybe.

THERAPIST: But your boss and parents will continue to annoy you?

MICHAEL: Yeah, probably. And my sister.

THERAPIST: So would you like to have as a goal to learn how not to be annoyed so much? How not to let them make you feel small?

MICHAEL: Yeah, I guess that would be good.

In the excerpt above, the therapist ascertains that the patient's reaction to her is part of a larger pattern. She judges that it is worth spending time working out the problem in the therapeutic relationship because she will then have the opportunity to improve their alliance and help the patient generalize what he learned to other important relationships. Note how she facilitated the patient's agreement to make the problem into a goal by empathizing with his annoyance and offering him a way to feel better. In the excerpt below, the therapist offers an alternative viewpoint.

THERAPIST: So we could start with me. I guess you have a choice. When I say something positive or explain something too much or disagree with you, you could say, "[My therapist] is patronizing me," and then you'll feel annoyed, even if I genuinely was not trying to make you feel small . . . . Or you could say, "[My therapist] isn't trying to patronize me. She's trying to help me feel better" or "That's just her way." (*pause*) Or I suppose you could say, "Just because she thinks I didn't know something or she sincerely does think this small thing I did was good doesn't make me small. There *are* things I have to learn to get over this depression. And I do deserve credit for the things I do." (*pause*) What do you think?

MICHAEL: I don't know.

THERAPIST: Well, if you *were* able to tell yourself, "She's right—I do deserve credit." or "It's good that I already knew that," would you feel less annoyed?

MICHAEL: Yeah, I suppose so.

THERAPIST: Well, it's something to think about. Maybe we can talk more about it next week.

MICHAEL: Okay.

The therapist senses that the patient is not ready to adopt this more functional (and more accurate) perspective at the moment. She has planted a seed and will assess at succeeding sessions the degree to which they still need to directly work on this problem. Once the patient has indeed modified his perception of the therapist, she can help him transfer his new understanding about feeling patronized to other relationships and do a combination of assertiveness training (so that he can be appropriately assertive with others), and responding to his dysfunctional beliefs.

SUMMARY

Many patients with challenging problems respond well when therapists use or modify their use of standard cognitive therapy principles to build a strong therapeutic alliance. Other patients present a greater challenge. The difficulties they present, however, offer the therapist an opportunity to better conceptualize patients' dysfunctional beliefs and to gain insight into the effect of their behavior on others. The therapeutic relationship can be a powerful agent of change, as therapists help patients modify their negative view of themselves and of the therapist, and then apply their learning to modify negative ideas about other people.

CHAPTER 5

Therapeutic Relationship Problems
Case Examples

The following case examples illustrate common difficulties that can arise in the therapeutic relationship. The first few examples illustrate patients who become angry at their therapists for a variety of reasons: they believe the therapist invalidated them, was about to reject them, was trying to control them, did not understand them, or did not care about them. Then examples are presented of patients who are skeptical about treatment, feel coerced into treatment, or resist the structure of treatment. The next set of examples depict a patient who provides negative feedback at the end of a session and a patient who fails to give negative feedback to the therapist, even when warranted. Finally, there is an example of a patient who avoids revealing important information to the therapist.

CASE EXAMPLE 1: THE PATIENT WHO FELT INVALIDATED BY THE THERAPIST

In one particular session, Rosalind described a situation in which she felt invalidated by her brother's treatment of her. When her therapist started to question her perception, she began to feel invalidated. The therapist conceptualized the difficulty, then changed his strategy.

THERAPIST: (*summarizing*) So when David [Rosalind's brother] said he wouldn't change his family's plans, you thought, "There he goes again, never accommodating *me* and *my* family, always doing what *he* wants to do." And you felt really hurt and angry. (*pause*) Is that right?

ROSALIND: Yeah. He *never* considers my feelings, never thinks about how what *he* does affects *me*!

THERAPIST: And what does that mean? Or what's the worst part about that?

ROSALIND: It means I'm not important.

THERAPIST: Is there any other explanation for why he didn't want to change his plans—other than that he thinks you're not important and doesn't care?

ROSALIND: You don't understand! He's always been that way! He always puts himself first!

THERAPIST: Oh, it sounds as if he's the most important one in his own eyes, then.

ROSALIND: Well, yeah!

THERAPIST: And that's very hurtful to you.

ROSALIND: Yeah.

THERAPIST: I'd like to see if we can help you feel less distressed by this. Would that be okay?

ROSALIND: (*angrily*) Are you saying I shouldn't be distressed? That's what people always say! You're like everyone else! You just don't get it!

THERAPIST: (*calmly*) Well, you may be right that I don't get it, but I *wasn't* saying that you shouldn't be distressed. Given what you were thinking, you should be!

ROSALIND: So now you're saying that my *thinking* was wrong.

THERAPIST: Actually, I don't know—you may be 100% correct. All I know for *sure* is that you're very upset about your brother—and I'd like to see if we can do something to make you feel less upset. (*pause*) But is there something bad about trying to feel less upset?

ROSALIND: It's like you're saying I'm wrong. Like everyone else (*mimicking*) "Rosalind, you're overreacting," "Rosalind, you're too sensitive."

The therapist realizes that he has to change gears. Trying to investigate whether her brother might have had other motives activated Rosalind's ideas of being misunderstood and being viewed as wrong and flawed. The therapist truly did not at that point know to what degree the patient had been accurate in her assessment of her brother. And he cannot know until they jointly examine the evidence and perhaps consider alternative explanations for his behavior. However, the therapist judges that doing so at this point would probably rupture their alliance. Instead the therapist empathizes with Rosalind, then decides to identify the belief underlying Rosalind's distressing reaction to her brother.

THERAPIST: Oh, that's a terrible way to feel. (*pause*) Let's assume that you're 100% right, that you *are* unimportant to your brother. What does that mean to you? . . . What's the worst part of that?

ROSALIND: (*settling down*) You see, I've always been pushed aside by my family. My parents, they have always favored my brother. He's the favorite. He's the golden boy. He got all the attention. They thought he walked on water. They *still* do.

THERAPIST: No wonder it's so hurtful. What does it mean to you that they and he do these things to you?

ROSALIND: Well, it makes me feel like I'm nothing [core belief].

THERAPIST: (*Nods.*) Nothing. (*pause*) Does this sound familiar? Seems to me we've talked about this idea before.

ROSALIND: Yeah.

Next they discuss whether Rosalind indeed really *was* nothing if she was ill-treated—or whether she was an important person regardless of her family's behavior. The therapist helped Rosalind identify her general assumptions: "If people don't accommodate me, it means they think I'm unimportant" and "If people think I'm unimportant, they're right—I'm nothing." The therapist asked Rosalind to continue to let him know if she ever felt that he was not treating her well, so they could solve the problem on the spot. At another session, the therapist helped Rosalind see that she was hypervigilant for others' treating her badly—and sometimes misinterpreted others' motives—because Rosalind herself felt as if she was "nothing."

CASE EXAMPLE 2: THE PATIENT WHO FEARED THE THERAPIST WOULD REJECT HER

Andrea's core belief was that she was bad. She was convinced that her therapist would also view her in an extremely negative light. Toward the end of their very first therapy session Andrea angrily told her therapist that she believed he would reject her. Her therapist responded in a direct, empathic, reassuring manner.

ANDREA: Why did you agree to see me [as a patient]? You'll probably get sick of me and throw me out of therapy like my other therapists.

THERAPIST: (*empathically*) Oh, you must have had *such* a hard time in the past. (*pause*) I'm sorry you had those experiences.

ANDREA: But you'll probably do the same thing.

THERAPIST: You know, I don't see that happening. I don't think I've ever actually *fired* a patient. Let me think. . . . There *have* been a few patients where we've *mutually* decided that they should try someone else . . . though I don't know why that would happen with you.

ANDREA: It probably will, though.

THERAPIST: What makes you think that? Have you picked up something about me?

ANDREA: You're a therapist. You're really all the same.

In the next part of the session, the therapist first acknowledges that the patient could be correct, then he helps the patient evaluate her thought ("You're really all the same") by differentiating himself and the treatment from the patient's previous therapeutic experiences.

THERAPIST: I guess that's *possible*, that I am the same. On the other hand, I have a pretty good track record of being able to help people who have tried other therapists.

ANDREA: (*changing the argument*) This therapy won't help anyway.

THERAPIST: What makes you think that? [a variation of "What's the evidence for this idea?"]

ANDREA: None of my previous therapy helped. I'm still depressed. My life is still lousy.

THERAPIST: (*referring to elements of cognitive therapy discussed earlier in the session*) Well, no wonder you don't have much confidence in therapy. (*pause*) Does it sound as if there is anything *different* about this therapy? Has every other therapist set an agenda with you, sent you home with therapy notes to read, asked you to give him feedback at the end of every session?

ANDREA: (*slowly*) . . . No.

THERAPIST: Well, actually that's hopeful. If I were planning to do *exactly* what your other therapists have done, I would say there's probably less of a chance that I can be helpful to you. (*pause*) I can't *guarantee* that I can help you, but I don't see any *reason* that I couldn't. (*pause*) Would you be willing to give this a chance for, say, four or five sessions—to see what happens?

ANDREA: I don't know if I can promise that.

THERAPIST: Then I guess we'll just have to go session by session for now. (*pause*) Meanwhile, it's *so* important that you told me that you think I'll throw you out of therapy. I need for you to *keep* letting me know when you have that thought. Would that be all right?

ANDREA: I suppose so. (*changing the subject*) I know you must think I'm a pain, you know, giving you a hard time and everything.

THERAPIST: (*providing as honestly positive a response as he can*) No, I *don't* think you're a pain. I think I understand why this is hard for you.

ANDREA: But your other patients . . . they must be easier.

THERAPIST: Well, yes, I guess some of them are. But that doesn't mean I don't want to keep working with you. (*implying that she is special*) You're *not* an everyday, garden-variety patient. You keep me on my toes.

Next the therapist checks on how much Andrea trusts his honesty:

THERAPIST: How much do you believe me when I say that I want to keep working with you?

ANDREA: (*looks away*) I don't know.

THERAPIST: (*guessing low*) 10%? 25%?

ANDREA: Maybe 25%.

THERAPIST: Okay, that's a good start. Well, time will tell, I guess. I want to repeat, though, that I don't want *you* to fire *me* as a therapist. I'd like to keep working with you.

During this interchange, Andrea's therapist conceptualized that Andrea's core belief of being bad and her assumption that others were likely to reject her became activated. He tried to differentiate himself and the therapy from Andrea's past therapists and therapeutic experiences and expressed a desire to keep treating Andrea. He sought, but did not insist upon from Andrea, a commitment to continue treatment, and reinforced Andrea for expressing her fears. He subtly reminded Andrea that he, the therapist, did not call all the shots and that *Andrea* had the power to end treatment if she wanted to. Doing these things calmed Andrea down and she did return for a full course of therapy.

CASE EXAMPLE 3: THE PATIENT WHO FELT CONTROLLED BY THE THERAPIST

Difficulties in the therapeutic alliance arose in the second therapy session with Jason, a 59-year-old man, as he and his therapist discussed how Jason might be able to improve his mood by changing his behavior. Jason became annoyed with his therapist's suggestion. The therapist chose to immediately demonstrate her willingness to go along with the patient because his prickliness in their first session led her to predict that he would react poorly at this point to her addressing the alliance issue directly.

THERAPIST: Do you think it would help if you tried getting out for a little while everyday?

JASON: (*flatly*) No!

THERAPIST: Then let's cross that off. Can you think of anything else you've done in the past that seemed to help lift your mood, even if was only a little?

A similar problem arose a few minutes later in the session. Hypothesizing that these two situations represented a dysfunctional pattern, the therapist directly addressed the issue. In the following transcript, Jason relates an ongoing pain problem.

THERAPIST: Have you considered asking your doctor again for help [with your migraines]?

JASON: No.

THERAPIST: Do you think it might be a good idea?

JASON: No!

THERAPIST: (*gently*) Jason, what went through your mind when I suggested that?

JASON: You're expecting me to work on the migraine problem and I don't want to take medicine—which won't work anyway—so there's really nothing I can do!

THERAPIST: (*showing surprise*) Jason, I'm confused. . . . What did you hear me say?

JASON: Well, you said I should work on my migraines—which means taking medicine. I'm already on way too much stuff!

THERAPIST: This is really important. I *don't* want you to work on your migraine problem now if it's going to cause you a lot of stress. (*pause*) Do you remember what I *actually* said?

JASON: Something about getting medication. But I don't want to do that!

THERAPIST: Then you shouldn't. And I'm sorry you're feeling distressed by this. But you need to know that I *don't* necessarily think you should automatically go on medication. When you're ready, you might just want to get more *information* from your doctor about your options. I *don't* necessarily think you should work on the migraines right now.

JASON: (*changing the subject*) It seems like everything we talk about is just a drop in the bucket.

THERAPIST: Well, you're right, in a sense. (*providing an analogy*] It is important for you to take small steps so you don't get overwhelmed . . . . But small steps everyday eventually can lead to a very long distance. And filling the bucket everyday with drops eventually fills it up.

JASON: (*Sighs.*)

THERAPIST: It doesn't sound as if what we've been talking about today has helped. Do you have a sense of what would help more?

JASON: (*Shakes his head.*)

THERAPIST: You know, I have the sense that we're on opposite sides of the fence. Do you have any ideas about how we can both get on the same side?

JASON: (*Shrugs.*)

THERAPIST: (*hypothesizing*) I'm wondering if you feel as if I don't really understand you, what things are like for you, that somehow I'm criticizing you or blaming you.

JASON: (*Mutters.*) Yeah.

THERAPIST: Maybe being so problem-solving oriented just won't work today. Maybe I should just listen more and try to understand.

JASON: (*pause*) I don't know.

THERAPIST: What do you think of *not* trying to move ahead today in terms of improving your life. (*pause*) Instead, maybe you could help me understand better what's going on with you.

JASON: (*Shrugs.*)

THERAPIST: Do you have the sense that I *want* to help?

JASON: I guess so.

THERAPIST: Well, you're right. I do.

JASON: But it *doesn't* help when you put all these expectations on me.

THERAPIST: Good to know. Okay, I'll make you a deal. I'll try not to put expectations on you today. But if you feel like I am, like you did with the meds, would you be willing to let me know? Then I'll tell you honestly whether I *did* make a mistake and did expect something. . . . What do you say?

JASON: (*slowly*) Okay.

THERAPIST: So, tell me, what don't I understand?

Jason had been feeling vulnerable and weak in the session. Hypervigilant for signs of being controlled and harmed, he jumped to conclusions about the therapist, mildly attacking her. His therapist responded calmly, corrected his misperception, and tried to provide hope when

Jason felt hopeless and denigrated the treatment. Recognizing a rupture in the therapeutic alliance, the therapist demonstrated her understanding by hypothesizing why the patient was feeling distressed, then offered to change what they were doing. The therapist indicated her desire to help the patient. She asked Jason to correct her in the future, trying to allow Jason to feel as if he were in the superior position. By listening carefully and demonstrating empathic, accurate understanding, the therapist helped to decrease Jason's expectation of harm, thus reducing his tendency to use a coping strategy of attacking others before they attacked him. Toward the end of the session, Jason has calmed down. The therapist then works directly on the relationship.

THERAPIST: What do you think? Was this second part of the session better?

JASON: Yeah.

THERAPIST: How much do you believe me when I say that I will try not to expect too much from you?

JASON: I guess I believe that you'll try—but I'm not sure that you won't do it anyway.

THERAPIST: Well, you may be right. And what's the safeguard?

JASON: I don't know.

THERAPIST: I think we agreed that you would check it out with me—to see if I had made that mistake so I could fix it.

JASON: Okay.

THERAPIST: Can you tell me, though, what would be the worst possibility if I *did* have unreasonable expectations for you?

JASON: I'd feel like I had to do what you wanted.

THERAPIST: Or else . . .?

JASON: Or you'd say you wouldn't help me any more. (*Mutters.*) My last therapist did that.

THERAPIST: Then I think we'd better have another agreement, if it's okay with you. I would like to keep working with you for as long as I can be helpful to you, whether or not you can do what we've talked about.

JASON: Yeah . . ..

THERAPIST: (*redressing the balance of power*) And I'd like you to keep working with *me*—and check out my intentions if you have the feeling that somehow I'm not on your side.

JASON: (*Pauses.*) Okay.

Jason's therapist understood that Jason was fragile. His painful core beliefs were continually activated during the session, even though his therapist was acting reasonably. His therapist recognized that she had to strengthen the therapeutic alliance and help Jason feel safe—or risk having Jason unilaterally terminate treatment. Next the therapist asked Jason what he thought he could do to have a better week, rather than suggesting homework assignments herself.

CASE EXAMPLE 4: THE PATIENT WHO CLAIMED HER THERAPIST DID NOT UNDERSTAND HER

June was a 37-year-old, unmarried woman with an unsatisfying and low-paying job. She was quite jealous of people whom she perceived as being better off than she—and she felt inferior in their presence. At the beginning of their second session, her therapist asks her whether she had any more goals to add to her goal list.

June: (*in an annoyed voice*) Listen, I don't think you understand.

THERAPIST: I don't understand . . .?

JUNE: What this is like for me! . . . After all, you're a professional. You make a lot of money. You're married and have kids . . .. You have all these things. All the things I don't.

THERAPIST: (*empathically*) Ohhh, that must feel so unfair to you.

JUNE: It does! It is!

THERAPIST: You're right; it is. (*pause*) Can you tell me a little bit more about what I don't understand? I'd really like to be able to help you better.

JUNE: (*calming down slightly*) Everything is a struggle. I have all these money problems. I have no one in my life. I'm really lonely. My dysfunctional family is always on my back. I hate my job. . . . .

THERAPIST: (*empathically*) You really *do* have it tough. (*pause*) I can't promise that I can make it easier for you, but I'd like to try, if you're willing. (*pause*) Maybe what we should do is to pick *one* problem to work on today—but you'll have to fill me in, so I *can* understand better. (*pause*) Would that be okay?

JUNE: (*begrudgingly*) I suppose.

THERAPIST: Where would you like to start?

Reviewing her goal list made June more conscious of the problems she faced. She began comparing herself to her therapist, who truly did have an easier and much more fulfilling life than June. When this comparison activated her core belief of inferiority, June employed her usual coping strategy of blaming others. Her therapist reacted empathically, stated her desire to help, asked the patient for permission to become problem-solving oriented, and made it clear she did want to understand. The patient reluctantly agreed to focus on one problem. They were able to make some headway on this problem and the patient felt somewhat better. At the end of the session, the therapist returned to the therapeutic relationship problem.

THERAPIST: I want to get back to something we started talking about at the beginning of the session. I got the impression that it's hard for you to come talk to me each week. I wonder, do you think you're comparing yourself to me a lot?

JUNE: I suppose so.

THERAPIST: I'm sorry it distresses you. Do you have an idea of how we can solve that problem?

JUNE: I don't know if it *can* be solved.

THERAPIST: (*pause*) Well, I'd like to keep trying. *My* preference is for us to keep working together. I *do* think I have something to offer you—like what we talked about today—how to set limits with your father so he doesn't upset you so much.

JUNE: (*Looks down and mutters.*) I don't know.

THERAPIST: Do you want to think about it this week and we can talk more about it next week?

JUNE: I guess so.

THERAPIST: And I will, too. (*pause*) I'm glad. I don't want you to fire me before we have a chance to fix this.

In this part of the session, the therapist made it clear that she preferred to solve their relationship problem and was willing to expend some effort thinking about it between sessions. The therapist also made a mental note to see whether comparing herself to other people was generally a problem for the patient.

CASE EXAMPLE 5: THE PATIENT WHO BELIEVED HIS THERAPIST DID NOT CARE

Alexander, a 68-year-old man, became angry at his therapist when she ended their fourth session on time. The therapist elicited Alexander's specific belief about her and also a general belief about others. She guided Alexander in modifying the belief in the context of their thera-peutic relationship and helped Alexander apply what he had learned to relationships with a friend and with his family.

THERAPIST: I see we only have a couple of minutes left. What did you think about today's session?

ALEXANDER: (*panicky voice*) But, but I have this problem with my sister. [Alexander had not put this problem on the agenda or mentioned it earlier in the session.] She's gone back to her old ways, you know, it's not like when I first got out of the hospital. She was so supportive then. But now . . .

THERAPIST: (*interrupting*) Oh, I'm sorry we don't have time to talk about that now. Can we put it first thing on the agenda to talk about next week?

ALEXANDER: But you don't understand, I really don't know what to do!

THERAPIST: I'm *really* sorry that we're out of time. I can see how upset you are by this. Do you want to schedule an earlier appointment so we can talk about it sooner?

ALEXANDER: No! I want to talk about it now!

THERAPIST: You must feel really let down, then. I promise you, though, that we'll talk about it first thing next week—and we'll also talk about my letting you down. Would that be okay?

ALEXANDER: (*Mutters angrily.*) I guess I don't have any choice.

THERAPIST: I'm sorry you're upset by this. You know what? Would you like to write me something about this and leave it for me with the recep-tionist? I'll read it before our next session and that'll give me some idea of what we should do.

ALEXANDER: (*in an annoyed voice*) Well, I won't write anything but I'll *tell* you next session.

THERAPIST: That's fine.

ALEXANDER: (*mutters*) Okay.

At the next session, Alexander's therapist immediately brings up the problem.

THERAPIST: Alexander, before we do anything else, can we talk about what happened at the end of the last session? What was most upset-ting to you?

ALEXANDER: Well, I had this really big problem and you obviously didn't want to hear about it.

THERAPIST: If it were true that I didn't, what would that mean?

ALEXANDER: You're only concerned with sticking to your time schedule.

THERAPIST: And if that were true, what would that mean?

ALEXANDER: You don't care about me. The schedule overrides everything.

THERAPIST: Well, I'm glad that you told me. Because it's really important to find out whether I do care about you or not.

ALEXANDER: Well, obviously, you don't.

THERAPIST: Okay, that's one possibility for why I ended the session on time—that I don't care anything about you or your problems. (*Writes it down.*) What's another possibility for why I ended the session on time?

ALEXANDER: I don't know.

THERAPIST: See, it's important for you to have all the facts before you make up your mind, especially about something that is going to cause you so much distress. (*pause*) The reason I need to end my therapy sessions on time is so I can finish writing up the important things about your session and anything I think we should do at our next session. Then I get out the file for my next patient, just as I did a few minutes ago with yours, so I could look at my notes and try to figure out how I can help the most.

ALEXANDER: I still think that if you really cared, you would have made the time.

THERAPIST: Are there any other ways that I've shown you that I care?

ALEXANDER: (*Looks down.*) I guess.

THERAPIST: How can you tell? (*offering evidence*) My tone of voice, when I say how sorry I am that you're so upset, (*pause*) when I work hard to help you solve problems?

ALEXANDER: I guess.

THERAPIST: Because I suppose I could just sit and listen and not say much and never make any effort to help.

ALEXANDER: Yeah. (*pause*) But if you *really* cared you'd give me the extra time.

THERAPIST: What else would I do if I really cared?

ALEXANDER: You'd let me call you between sessions, even if I weren't suicidal.

THERAPIST: Anything else?

ALEXANDER: (*Thinks.*) You'd tell my sister that she has to be nicer to me.

THERAPIST: (*writing these things down*) Anything else?

ALEXANDER: I don't know.

THERAPIST: And the fact that I'm not doing all these things means I don't care?

ALEXANDER: Well, if someone really cares, they give you 100%.

THERAPIST: Ohhhhh, I think I get it now. And if someone doesn't give 100%, it means . . . ?

ALEXANDER: That they don't care.

THERAPIST: Well, *no wonder* you had the idea I didn't care.

Next they discuss Alexander's dichotomous thinking—someone cares 100% and gives 100% or she does not care at all.

THERAPIST: What would happen if I *did* give you 100%? Would I be able to schedule any other patients? After all, you might want to talk to me at any time of the day or night. Would I be able to do what I needed to do at home? Would it even be *possible* for me to give you 100%?

ALEXANDER: (*slowly*) I suppose not.

THERAPIST: So *is* it possible, that even though I'm not giving you 100%, that I still care about you?

ALEXANDER: I'm not sure. (*pause*)

THERAPIST: Is there *anyone* who gives you 100%?

ALEXANDER: (*Thinks.*) No.

THERAPIST: Whom do you think cares about you the most?

ALEXANDER: My friend Nadine, I guess.

THERAPIST: Does *she* give you 100%?

ALEXANDER: No.

THERAPIST: Do you ever think *she* doesn't care?

ALEXANDER: Yeah, sometimes.

THERAPIST: When was the last time?

ALEXANDER: A couple of days ago. We were supposed to go out to dinner and at the last minute she said she had to work and couldn't go.

THERAPIST: And did you think, "Nadine doesn't care about me"?

ALEXANDER: Yeah. I mean if she did, she might have been able to get out of it. I know she's done that before.

THERAPIST: Do you see it any differently now?

ALEXANDER: I'm not sure.

THERAPIST: Could Nadine really give you 100% and still take care of herself?

ALEXANDER: I guess not.

THERAPIST: Do *you* care about *Nadine*?

ALEXANDER: Yeah, that's why it hurts so much when she does things like that.

THERAPIST: Do you give Nadine 100%?

ALEXANDER: (*long pause*) I guess not.

THERAPIST: How can that be, though? If you really cared about Nadine, wouldn't you rearrange your life so you could give her 100%?

ALEXANDER: (*Thinks.*) No. I guess I couldn't do that.

THERAPIST: So maybe this formula you have in your head isn't quite right? That you can care for people, yet not give them 100%? And that people could care for you, yet not give you 100%?

ALEXANDER: Maybe.

THERAPIST: So is it possible that *I* could care about you, even if I don't give you extra time?

ALEXANDER: (*slowly*) I guess so.

THERAPIST: But if you *assume* I don't care, what happens?

ALEXANDER: I get angry.

THERAPIST: Yeah, I hate to see you upset like that.

ALEXANDER: (*Sighs.*) But I *wish* you would give me more.

THERAPIST: Of course. And it must be hard for you that I'm not. But can you see that maybe I *do* care and that there are reasons that have nothing to do with caring for why I'm not giving you more?

ALEXANDER: Yeah.

THERAPIST: So what do you think would help for you to remind yourself this week?

The patient and therapist discuss an adaptive response. Alexander writes,

> [My therapist] can't give me 100%. That doesn't mean she doesn't care. In fact, she says she does and most of the time acts like she does. If I tell myself she doesn't care, I'll get really upset and it may not even be true.

THERAPIST: That's great. Now tell me, does this same card also apply to Nadine?

ALEXANDER: (*Sighs.*) Yeah.

THERAPIST: Do you want to add her name to the card, too, then?

ALEXANDER: Okay. (*Does so.*)

THERAPIST: One last thing—what we've talked about today—does it apply to anyone else, besides Nadine and me?

ALEXANDER: Ummm, maybe. I'm not sure. Maybe my sister.

THERAPIST: So when you read the card at home this week, can you see whether it applies to her?

ALEXANDER: Yeah.

At future sessions they discuss the belief that underlies the assumption. Alexander believes that he is at heart unlovable. Therefore, he is hypervigilant for people not caring—because their non-caring behavior demonstrates to him that he is unlovable. They also discuss another strategy Alexander has: reacting angrily and rejecting people first, before they can reject him.

CASE EXAMPLE 6: THE PATIENT WHO WAS SKEPTICAL ABOUT THERAPY

David had sought treatment from a number of mental health professionals before he started cognitive therapy treatment. He tended to drop out of therapy prematurely and had made little progress to date. He came to the first session feeling skeptical. In addition, when his therapist described the importance of learning to respond to his automatic thoughts, his core belief of incompetence became activated, and he employed his usual coping strategy of avoidance—in this case, perhaps by avoiding therapy altogether:

THERAPIST: Could you just summarize what we've been talking about?

DAVID: Well, I guess you were saying that I have to catch my depressed thinking and think more realistically. But, you know, I'm not sure this therapy is really for me. I don't think it's going to work. (*pause*) I just don't see how coming in and talking about my thinking will help.

THERAPIST: Well, you're right. Just coming in and talking *isn't* likely to help—or help *enough*. It's making small changes in your everyday life that will help.

DAVID: (*pause*) Maybe.

THERAPIST: Look, I think it's *good* that you're skeptical. You *shouldn't* just take my word for it. You'll need to try things out and see what happens—see whether the things we talk about in session and the things you try at home make you feel better or not. (*pause*) Is there something *specifically* about the therapy or about me that makes you think it won't work?

DAVID: This automatic thought stuff. I don't know if it applies to me.

THERAPIST: Well, I guess if you're willing to come back for the next couple of weeks we can figure that out together. (*pause*) Is it that you don't think you *have* automatic thoughts—or are you thinking you do have them but you might not be able to answer them back and feel better?

DAVID: The second, I guess.

THERAPIST: Well, that's *my* job. You *shouldn't* know how to answer them back yet. You've never *been* in this kind of therapy before. We'll just take it step by step—and you'll let me know if I'm helping you enough or not. Fair enough?

DAVID: Yeah.

The therapist was careful to acknowledge the patient's skepticism. She reduced his anxiety by asking him to return for only 2 more weeks and by taking responsibility for his making progress. He then settled down and was able to work more collaboratively with her.

CASE EXAMPLE 7: THE PATIENT WHO FELT COERCED INTO THERAPY

Roger, a 16-year-old adolescent, was mandated by his school and parents to get treatment. Like many other patients who enter therapy at the insistence of others, he was quite unhappy to be in a therapist's office. His therapist hypothesized about his automatic thoughts and empathized with and normalized his reaction, then tried to demonstrate the advantages therapy could have for him.

THERAPIST: So what problem do you want help with today?

ROGER: (*Looks away.*)

THERAPIST: Well, what's been bothering you lately? Your family, school, other kids?

ROGER: (*Looks irritated and does not answer.*)

THERAPIST: You know, if I were in your position, this office is about the *last* place I'd want to be. I'll bet it wasn't *your* idea to come here.

ROGER: No.

THERAPIST: And if I were you, I'd be thinking, "Why should I talk to this woman? She doesn't know me. She probably thinks she can help but she can't." (*pause*) Am I close?

ROGER: I guess so.

THERAPIST: And I'd be thinking, "What do I have to do to get out of here? I hate this." (*pause*) Am I right?

ROGER: (*sighs*) I don't know.

THERAPIST: Well, let me say outright: I don't know if I can help you or not. And I don't blame you for not wanting to be here . . ..But as long as you *are* here, I'd like to see if I can help . . ..Of course, *you'll* have to be the judge of that—whether it's been worth talking to me or I'm a total flop.

ROGER: (*Looks surprised.*)

THERAPIST: So as long as you're here, can you tell me what you wish were different in your life? (*pause*) For example, do you wish your parents would get off your back?

ROGER: I guess.

THERAPIST: Anyone else on your back? Teachers? Other kids?

ROGER: (*in a disgusted voice*) Teachers. I wish they'd leave me alone.

THERAPIST: Okay, Two problems. (*writing them down*) Parents. Teachers . . .. Now before we begin, if you feel like your parents and teachers are on your back, you may start to feel as if *I'm* on your back, too. So it's really important to let me know if you ever think I am. (*pause*) Because otherwise this therapy isn't going to work. (*pause*) Would you be willing to tell me if I ever sound like your parents or your teachers?

ROGER: I guess.

THERAPIST: Good. Now what do you want to talk about first, your family or school?

Roger's therapist had to differentiate herself from other adults in Roger's life and state outright that she did not want to control him as he correctly perceived his parents and teachers did. Her stance surprised Roger. He was then able to differentiate his therapist from the others and was a little more willing to collaborate.

CASE EXAMPLE 8: THE PATIENT WHO GAVE NEGATIVE FEEDBACK

Meredith's therapist had failed to pick up her discomfort during a session and had not left sufficient time at the end of the session to respond to her negative feedback. The therapist reinforced Meredith for expressing her distress and made it clear that he wanted to address the difficulty in their next session.

THERAPIST: Was there anything you didn't like about the session or anything you thought I got wrong or didn't understand?

MEREDITH: Well, yes, actually. I really don't appreciate it when you keep making me tell you how much I believe something or how much I feel some emotion. I hate having to measure stuff on a scale.

THERAPIST: I'm sorry that distresses you, but I'm really glad you told me. Would it be all right if we solve this first thing next week? (*Writes it down on therapy note.*) I wish we had time to talk about it right now but actually I would like to think about it this week. I don't want to just give you a flip answer. So if it's okay with you, we'll take it up before we talk about anything else at our next session. Would that be all right?

MEREDITH: Yeah, I guess so.

THERAPIST: Is there anything else that bothered you about the session?

MEREDITH: No, I guess not.

At the following session, Meredith's therapist repeated the rationale for asking Meredith to measure her degree of belief and emotions. They agreed that the therapist could probably find out enough to help Meredith by asking for her assessment in more general terms: "Do you believe that a little, a medium amount, a lot?"; "Do you feel better, the same, or worse right now?"

Meredith's prickliness showed up in many different situations in treatment, giving her therapist many opportunities to model interpersonal problem solving, which strengthened the therapeutic alliance. Her therapist soon recognized that Meredith reacted irritably whenever her core belief of incompetence became activated—both in session and out. Initially the therapist tried to avoid its activation in session, focusing on helping Meredith solve problems and adaptively respond to thoughts with the theme of incompetence about situations *outside* of therapy (paying her bills, hiring repairmen for her home, buying a used computer). Then she helped Meredith apply what she had learned from solving these problems to situations in which she felt incompetent in session.

CASE EXAMPLE 9: THE PATIENT WHO AVOIDED GIVING HONEST FEEDBACK TO THE THERAPIST

Sheila's therapist suspected that Sheila had had an unexpressed negative reaction to their therapy session. At the end of the session, the therapist encouraged her to give honest feedback.

THERAPIST: This session was a little different today. It felt like I was pushing you a lot. Did it seem that way to you, too?

SHEILA: No, not really. I know you're just trying to help.

THERAPIST: Do you feel like we're going too fast [with your agoraphobic hierarchy]?

SHEILA: (*slowly*) No, I guess not. I mean I know I just have to do these things or I won't get better.

THERAPIST: If you did feel like I was pushing too hard, would you be able to let me know?

SHEILA: I think so.

THERAPIST: That's good, because I want to make sure that we make this therapy right for you. If you start thinking differently about this at home, would you be sure to let me know at the beginning of our next session?

Sheila's therapist was careful to give her permission to give him negative feedback and to imply that he was willing to change what they were doing, if need be. Failure to demonstrate this kind of openness and flexibility can sometimes lead to patients' abrupt withdrawal from therapy.

CASE EXAMPLE 10: THE PATIENT WHO AVOIDED REVEALING IMPORTANT INFORMATION

Mandy appeared quite nervous in session because she predicted her therapist's questioning would lead her to reveal the physical abuse her mother had heaped upon her when she was a child. Mandy was wringing her hands and her face looked worried and drawn. When her therapist questioned Mandy about her thoughts, she looked down and whispered, "I can't tell you." Her therapist judged that their alliance was strong enough to push her a little:

THERAPIST: Well, that's okay, but can you tell me, are you feeling anxious?

MANDY: Yeah.

THERAPIST: You don't have to tell me what was going through your mind, but could you tell me what you're afraid could happen if you *did* tell me?

MANDY: (*still whispering and looking down*) You might think I was bad. You might not want to see me any more.

THERAPIST: (*summarizing matter of factly in the form of the cognitive model*) So the situation is that I asked you what you were thinking, and you had the automatic thought, "If I tell [my therapist], she might think I'm bad. She might not want to see me any more," and those thoughts made you feel anxious. Is that right?

MANDY: Yes.

THERAPIST: Well, you don't have to tell me what you were thinking, but could we look at these thoughts: "[My therapist] will think I'm bad. She might not want to see me any more?"

MANDY: (*Nods.*)

THERAPIST: Do you have some *evidence* that I'll think you're bad and won't want to see you any more?

MANDY: (*Curls up in chair.*) Well, what happened was really bad.

THERAPIST: (*offering an alternative view*) Is it possible that *I* won't see it as bad? (*pause*) Or even if I do, that I wouldn't see *you* as a wholly bad person?

MANDY: (*whispering*) I guess so.

THERAPIST: Do you have any evidence on the other side—that maybe I won't think harshly of you at all? That maybe I *will* want to keep seeing you?

MANDY: I don't know.

THERAPIST: Have you told me any bad things before?

MANDY: I don't know.

THERAPIST: Well, what about the problem with your sister? Do you remember that you were also afraid that I would see you as bad?

MANDY: (*Nods.*)

THERAPIST: And how did I react? Was I disapproving?

MANDY: (*in a quiet voice, still not making eye contact*) No.

THERAPIST: Are you sure?

MANDY: Yeah.

THERAPIST: So how did I seem?

MANDY: You were actually on my side. You said you thought she was being unreasonable.

THERAPIST: Right. (*Lets that sink in.*) Now, what's the worst that could happen if I *did* see you as bad?

MANDY: You wouldn't want me to keep being your patient.

THERAPIST: Okay, that's the worst. (*pause*) What's the best that could happen?

MANDY: I don't know. I guess that you would want me to keep coming.

THERAPIST: And what's the most realistic scenario?

MANDY: (*Thinks.*) Maybe that you'll think I am bad but you'll still be willing to see me?

THERAPIST: Or maybe I'll see you as *human*, not as bad?

MANDY: I don't know. (*pause*)

THERAPIST: Do you want to tell me just one small part of it and see how I react? Then you could decide whether or not to tell me more.

MANDY: I guess so.

When Mandy was too anxious to reveal her thoughts, her therapist instead elicited Mandy's fears about revealing her thoughts. She helped Mandy evaluate her predictions in a matter-of-fact way, and provided an alternative viewpoint—which helped the patient realize that her negative predictions might not come true. Her therapist offered her the option of revealing just a small part. Mandy then revealed an incident from childhood in which her mother physically abused her. Her therapist showed sympathy and caring. Mandy began to believe less strongly that her therapist would judge her negatively and reject her and she was willing to reveal more.

SUMMARY

The patients depicted in the case examples in this chapter have a particularly hard time developing an alliance with their therapists. Most patients do not present such significant difficulties. However, it is important to be prepared for the variety of ways in which the therapeutic relationship may be tested and strained. It is vital for therapists to remain calm and nondefensive. When difficulties arise, they need to conceptualize problems and determine whether patients are feeling vulnerable, coerced, controlled, invalidated, or rejected. Therapists can express understanding and empathy, and then carefully begin to engage patients in evaluating the therapeutic relationship as objectively and constructively as possible. Therapists need to bring the best of their own interpersonal skills to bear on the problem, modeling honesty, openness, flexibility, and optimism in repairing the therapeutic relationship so that therapy can progress. When they have difficulty doing so, they may need to adjust their own attitudes and behavior, as described in the next chapter.

CHAPTER 6

When Therapists Have Dysfunctional Reactions to Patients

By virtue of being human, therapists sometimes have attitudes regarding patients (especially those with challenging problems) that can interfere with therapy. Therapists who expect that such attitudes may arise naturally from time to time and who do not blame themselves unduly are usually able to take a problem-solving approach to resolve the difficulty. Therapists who hold unrealistically high expectations ("I should never feel negatively toward a patient") and who criticize themselves for having negative reactions ("This shows I'm a bad therapist") are likely to face a greater challenge in solving the problem (Leahy, 2001).

Having identified a dysfunctional reaction, the therapist must try to solve the problem. As with most therapeutic challenges, the issue may be practical (e.g., the therapist is feeling overburdened because he has not set appropriate limits with the patient), psychological (e.g., the therapist has interfering beliefs such as "My patients should appreciate me") or both. Finally, therapists need to monitor their own level of self-care to make sure that they are in good shape to help their patients. Identifying and solving problems in therapists' reactions to patients is presented first in the chapter, followed by case examples illustrating typical difficulties.

IDENTIFYING PROBLEMS IN THERAPISTS' REACTIONS

Therapists can usually pick up on their own negative reactions to patients by noticing a change in their thinking, emotions, behavior, or physiology (unless their reactions are mild or chronic). Some changes, though, may be too subtle for therapists to recognize—for example, shifts in their tone of voice, body language or facial expression. A quick way for therapists to assess whether they are having negative reactions to their patients is to monitor their thoughts and feelings as they review the list of patients they are scheduled to see on a given day. Feelings of discomfort are a warning signal that therapists need to examine their reaction and respond adaptively to their thoughts so that they can both feel and project a positive attitude toward the patient. A useful question for therapists to ask themselves is:

> ■ "Who do I wish would cancel his/her session today?"

If therapists can identify patients who fall into this category, they should consider the need to prepare differently for them, and perhaps to change their therapeutic strategies.

On an ongoing basis, therapists need to assess their overall level of empathy for a patient. And they need to monitor their reactions—any changes in emotional, behavioral, or physiological response—just before, during, and after sessions, by asking themselves:

> ■ "Do I feel annoyed, angry, anxious, sad, hopeless, overwhelmed, guilty, embarrassed, demeaned?"
> ■ "Am I engaging in any dysfunctional behaviors, such as blaming, dominating, or controlling the patient? Or am I being too passive?"
> ■ "Is my volume/tone of voice, facial expression, body language appropriate?"
> ■ "Am I feeling tense? is my heart beating faster? Is my face becoming hot?"

Patients often recognize these kinds of changes in their therapists—which can lead to a rupture in the alliance. Sometimes patients perceive these changes accurately (Henry correctly picks up his therapist's hopelessness) and sometimes inaccurately (Pam misreads her therapist's anxiety concerning his own adequacy as annoyance with her). These changes usually indicate that therapists are having automatic thoughts about the patient or about themselves that may need to be evaluated and addressed. Before sessions, for example, therapists may make predictions such as:

> ■ "[The patient] will:
>
>   be feeling worse
>   not make any progress
>   take too much energy
>   overwhelm me
>   blame me, argue with me, make me feel uncomfortable
>   be unappreciative
>   demand entitlements
>   expect me to solve all his problems
>   not let me do what I'm supposed to do."

Therapists may find themselves making the same kind of cognitive errors (about the patient or about themselves) that their patients make (Leahy, 1996).

Overgeneralizing and labeling
"Since [this patient] didn't do his homework, it shows he is lazy."
"I must be stupid to have missed the level of the patient's distress."
"Homework is useless with these kinds of patients."

Catastrophizing
"This patient will never get better."
"I'll never be able to get through to [this patient]."
"This patient is looking for a mistake so he/she can sue me!"

Disqualifying the positive
"While [this patient] did some of the homework, she's still not trying
    hard enough."
"Even though the patient is satisfied with his progress, I should be
    helping him so much more."
"Last week's progress was an illusion."

CONCEPTUALIZING NEGATIVE REACTIONS

It is important for therapists to use their own emotional reactions and dysfunctional behavior as signals to identify potential problems. When noticing their own discomfort or maladaptive behavior (e.g., avoiding important topics, overcontrolling or undercontrolling patients, speaking sharply or without empathy), therapists should identify their dysfunctional thoughts and beliefs and conceptualize their area of vulnerability. Some therapists, for example, feel overly responsible for solving all their patients' problems. Some feel out of control when their patients are deeply emotional or overly dominating in session. Some become angry at patients who continue to act dysfunctionally or who violate the therapist's morals.

To conceptualize their own dysfunctional emotional or behavioral reactions, therapists should ask themselves:

■ "What does it mean to me that [this patient] is engaging in this behavior?"
■ "What does it imply to me about the success of therapy?"
■ "What does it ultimately mean about me?"

Often therapists ascribe negative meanings to patients: "[This behavior means that] the patient is bad, weak, unworthy." Or they may ascribe negative meanings to themselves: ["The patient's failure to progress means that] I am inadequate, incompetent."

Case Example 1

When Harry described several interactions he had had with his son during the previous week, it became apparent to the therapist that Harry's behavior was terribly demeaning. Her initial reaction was to label Harry as an emotionally abusive parent and a bad person. She began to question whether she would be able to influence the patient enough to "save" the child. The therapist's sense of helplessness, rigid moral sensibility, and dysfunctionally strong sense of responsibility led her to feel anger and indignation and she began to blame the patient and to dominate him. Her attitudes and behavior interfered with her ability to help the patient control his anger with his son and learn more adaptive coping strategies.

Case Example 2

Mary began to weep as she described the maltreatment she had experienced as a child at the hands of her peers in the neighborhood. Her therapist catastrophized Mary's outpouring of emotion: "It's terrible that she is so upset! What if she keeps on crying? I have to get her to stop!" The therapist felt overwhelmed and incompetent to deal with his patient's distress. He abruptly, and noncollaboratively, changed the subject, leading the patient to view him as unempathic and unhelpful.

Case Example 3

A therapist was doing couple therapy with Craig, a man who was high powered and overcontrolling, and Amy, a woman who was meek and submissive. Whenever the therapist tried to interrupt Craig so she could elicit his wife's point of view, Craig became impatient with and dismissive of the therapist. The therapist, who frequently felt emotionally vulnerable herself, became anxious about prompting his irritation and avoided doing so, becoming too passive in session.

Case Example 4

Isabelle characteristically put others down in order to feel superior herself. When she belittled her therapist's suggestions, he first felt hurt, then angry. The therapist's beliefs about being weak and incompetent had been activated. In his *own* characteristic way, the therapist began to bully the patient, in an effort to redress the balance of power in the session.

STRATEGIES TO IMPROVE THERAPISTS' REACTIONS TO PATIENTS

Therapists can employ a number of strategies once they have conceptualized the problem they are experiencing in their reaction to patients. These strategies include:

- Increasing their competence.
- Responding to their cognitions.
- Developing realistic expectations for themselves and for their patients.
- Moderating their level and expression of empathy.
- Setting limits.
- Giving feedback to patients.
- Enhancing self-care.
- Transferring the patient to another clinician.

Increasing Therapist Competence

Sometimes therapists experience a negative reaction to a patient because they themselves simply lack important skills and need to increase their own competence in diagnosis, cognitive formulation and conceptualization, alliance building, treatment planning, developing overall strategy, structuring the session, or implementing techniques. This can be accomplished through reading, viewing master videotapes, or receiving additional training, consultation, or supervision. Appendix A offers an array of resources to improve therapist effectiveness.

Responding to Dysfunctional Cognitions

A critical part of ameliorating negative reactions to patients is responding to negative cognitions. Dysfunctional Thought Records (J. Beck, 2005) can be helpful. It may be useful to read alternative responses, such as those below, on a regular basis.

He's giving me a hard time because he's in a lot of emotional pain and this is the only way he knows of dealing with it. He has many really difficult problems and he'll need to be in therapy for a long time. I shouldn't expect him to change quickly and easily.

> She wants me to solve all her problems for her without having to change herself because she honestly believes she is too helpless to do anything to help herself.

> She's blocking my attempts to help her because she thinks if she gets better, her life will get worse. If I can't figure out how to solve this problem on my own, I can read or consult with others.

While the automatic thoughts of therapists who have patients with challenging problems are usually *negative*, some may be overly *positive*:

> - "This patient is special and should be treated specially."
> - "I want more than a therapeutic relationship with [this patient]."

When therapists do have overly positive reactions to patients, the therapeutic relationship may become too similar to a friendship with a consequent loss of sufficient focus on the patient's problems. Or therapists may have sexual feelings toward their patients, which they need to recognize and manage in a professionally responsible and ethical manner, so that therapy may proceed in a way that is beneficial for the patient (Pope, Sonne & Horoyd, 1993). Consultation in such situations can be quite helpful and is sometimes essential.

Developing Realistic Expectations for Oneself and for One's Patients

Therapists may or may not be fully cognizant of their expectations. When their expectations are too high or too low, therapists may develop maladaptive reactions. Sonia's therapist became frustrated because Sonia resisted looking for a full-time job; he had not yet realized just how symptomatic and dysfunctional Sonia became during her depressive and manic episodes. The expectations of Robert's therapist were too low; she overempathized with Robert's misfortunes and failed to gently push him toward change. Sandy's therapist had unrealistic expectations for himself, believing that he should be able to fix all of Sandy's problems, and became too anxious about his own performance and Sandy's slow progress.

Moderating One's Level and Expression of Empathy

In many cases, therapists need to increase their sense of empathy toward patients. It is important to conceptualize why patients are acting they way they are, by understanding how their early life experiences and genetic predisposition contributed to the development of negative beliefs about themselves, their worlds, and other people (including the therapist) and to the use of a small set of coping strategies (dysfunctional behaviors that they employ in therapy, too). It is also helpful to conceptualize at approximately what developmental level patients seem to be operating at difficult points during the therapy session. Many patients become quite childlike in their thinking, emotional reaction, or behavior. Perceiving the adult patient as a highly distressed child or adolescent can increase therapist empathy.

Case Example 5

For the first 3 months of therapy, Gary, age 25, was sometimes critical of or even demeaning to his therapist. She conceptualized that when Gary entered her office, he felt like a child again. He perceived that his therapist would put him down, just as his father, and many others in his life, had done while Gary was growing up. Gary was obviously not operating as a mature adult in session. He was like an 8-year-old boy, expecting to be demeaned, so he protected himself by putting his therapist down first.

In some cases, however, therapists are *overly* empathic with patients. Therapists may incorrectly believe that their patients' negative view of problems is entirely accurate or that their problems are insoluble. In some cases, too much direct expression of empathy can actually make patients feel worse.

Case Example 6

Connie, who had been chronically depressed for many years, had a very poor relationship with her husband and felt quite stuck and helpless. Her therapist, empathizing too much with Connie's distress, did not believe she was capable of standing up to her husband, learning new techniques to handle her recalcitrant teenage son, or pursuing interests outside of the house. Having consulted with a colleague, the therapist tested her assumptions and encouraged her patient to try some behavioral experiments. Indeed, Connie was able to make small differences in all three areas, which gave her hope and motivation to get unstuck in her life.

Case Example 7

Amy's therapist expressed too much empathy at times. When Amy became quite upset in session, her therapist kept saying how sorry she was that Amy had such difficult problems and felt so badly. The more her therapist empathized, the worse Amy felt. It was not until her therapist helped her to become problem-solving oriented that Amy began to feel better.

Setting Appropriate Limits

When patients take a great deal of therapists' time and energy, therapists sometimes begin to resent them. In such cases, therapists should assess whether they have set reasonable limits with their patients. They may, for example, have drifted into giving patients extra time in session, talking by phone with patients who are not in crisis, or promising to do some other special favor. Having recognized such a difficulty, therapists may need to put the problem on the agenda and do creative problem solving with patients. For example, if a patient is calling too often, she may need more frequent appointments (perhaps twice a week for half sessions instead of once a week for full sessions). Patients may respond negatively when therapists bring up such topics. The therapist must be prepared to correct patients' incorrect assumptions, such as "[My therapist] doesn't care about me."

Giving Feedback to Patients

Generally therapists do not bring up their own negative reactions to patients. When they do so, they should make sure beforehand that it is the *patient* who is behaving unreasonably and that they themselves are having a reasonable, though negative, reaction. They should have a strong rationale for relating their negative reaction: the intention is to improve the therapeutic alliance and to provide an important learning experience for patients so that they can also improve their relationships outside of therapy. Therapists need to watch their language carefully, so as not to sound critical, and choose an appropriate point in therapy, when the therapeutic alliance is sufficiently strong, before discussing a negative reaction. In the example below, the therapist discusses how she feels when she perceives the patient is manipulating her—though she does not use that pejorative term.

THERAPIST: I've noticed something about our therapy together that I wanted to talk to you about—because I think it could help you with your sister and your friend, Barbara, and your neighbor, Toby. Okay if I bring it up?

PATIENT: (*Shrugs.*)

THERAPIST: As I do, I want you to watch out for what you're thinking and how you're feeling—because I predict you might get mad at me. Okay?

PATIENT: Okay.

THERAPIST: And it will be important for you to tell me if you think I'm right about this or if I'm off-base. (*pause*) I've noticed I sometimes have to turn you down on things—like taking extra time in the session if you're late or letting you use my office phone. And when I say no, it feels to me as if you keep trying to persuade me or pressure me to change my mind. And then I start to feel a little resentful that you won't take no for an answer. (*pause*) Have you noticed anything like that?

PATIENT: I'm not sure.

THERAPIST: Well, the reason I wanted to bring it up is not so much for my sake—but I'm wondering whether other people might be reacting to you in the same way. Do you think this kind of thing might be happening with your sister or your friends? Do you think you might have trouble taking no for an answer? (*pause*) Maybe if we could figure out how to handle this here in therapy, you'd be able to act differently with other people, too. (*pause*) What do you think?

Similarly, therapists may choose to write a letter to their patients (and then ask them to read it in session), in which they carefully spell out the problems that need to be solved collaboratively in order to move forward in a healthy and productive way (Newman, 1997). Ideally, the letter should be an invitation to resume treatment in a spirit of teamwork, with mutual understanding and shared striving toward negotiated goals. Writing a letter allows therapists the opportunity to weigh their words carefully, thus potentially maximizing the value of the corrective feedback, while minimizing the chance of inadvertently inflaming the situation.

Enhancing Self-Care

Therapists should assess the degree to which they are practicing good *self-care* activities. If doing so is within their control, they can strategically schedule patients toward whom they may have a negative reaction. Making appointments with these patients at the beginning of the day or after a lunch break can give the therapist more time to mentally and emotionally prepare for the patient. Alternately, scheduling them just before lunch or at the end of the day allows the therapist time to immediately reflect on the session. In addition, therapists may need to change their overall home and work schedule if they are chronically rushed or overextended. Adding relaxation or mindfulness exercises to their daily routine may be useful.

Transferring the Patient

Therapists might consider discussing with the patient the possibility of transferring to another therapist when it appears that the advantages to the patient outweigh the disadvantages to the patient. A decision such as this should be made collaboratively. Sometimes a fresh start with a new therapist engenders hope, energy and a fresh perspective. It is important to have as positive an ending as possible with the patient, with the therapist expressing regret that he or she could not help the patient more and indicating confidence that the patient will progress better with a different clinician.

CASE EXAMPLES

The following case examples illustrate how to conceptualize and strategize when therapists have negative reactions to patients. Several situations are depicted: (1) when therapists feel hopeless about patients, (2) when therapists feel overburdened by patients, (3) when therapists believe they will displease patients, and (4) when therapists feel anxious, demeaned, defensive, frustrated, or threatened.

When Therapists Are Hopeless about Patients

Three problems often underlie this kind of negative reaction. Therapists may believe:

- "I am not competent enough to help [this patient]."
- "[The patient's] problems simply can't be solved."
- "[The patient] is experiencing a normal reaction to life stress and therefore there is nothing I can do to help."

Sometimes therapists feel incompetent because their expectations for their patients are too high.

Stacy's therapist labeled himself as inadequate when she failed to progress quickly. He started to feel hopeless about himself and his patient's prognosis ("I'm doing a lousy job—she's not going to get better"). He unknowingly transmitted his hopelessness to Stacy, who then became even more hopeless herself. Stacy's therapist needed consultation to recognize that he was in fact doing a reasonable job with his chronically depressed patient and that he needed to modify his (and the patient's) expectations for the pace of progress and length of treatment.

Sometimes therapists feel hopeless because their treatment actually *is* inadequate.

> Tyler suffered from obsessive–compulsive disorder (OCD). Unfamiliar with the specific guidelines for treating OCD with cognitive therapy, his therapist continued to treat Tyler as if he had generalized anxiety disorder. Tyler continued to be highly symptomatic, and his therapist felt increasingly hopeless. It was not until his therapist learned about and then implemented OCD treatment that the patient began to improve and the therapist's hopelessness decreased.

Sometimes therapists feel hopeless because they accept their patients' distorted view of their problems.

> Don was depressed and had multiple life problems and stressors: financial difficulties, health problems, a demanding boss, and a child with a chronic illness. His therapist thought, "He's not making progress because his problems aren't solvable," and felt hopeless. Her view led her to lapse back into providing only supportive psychotherapy, the modality in which she had originally been trained. She stopped trying to help Don solve problems or to teach him needed skills. When she finally sought supervision, her supervisor pointed out that while just about anyone in the patient's position would be distressed, not everyone would become clinically depressed. Therefore, the therapist should assume that Don had at least some maladaptive thoughts and beliefs that could be modified to help him feel better and that Don probably needed some help in problem solving. For example, like many depressed patients, Don had withdrawn from activities he had previous enjoyed and needed help from his therapist to figure out how to reengage in these activities.

When Therapists Feel Overburdened by Patients

Therapists may be overburdened due to practical problems: patients' illnesses, for example, may be too severe for the level of care they are receiving.

> Larry had bipolar disorder and required periodic hospitalization. He often called his therapist when he was in true crisis. Because of financial and insurance restraints, his therapist was seeing him only once a week even though Larry needed to be in a partial hospitalization program. His therapist helped Larry to apply for and receive Medicaid, and the patient was finally able to receive the appropriate level of care.

Often, however, therapists feel overburdened because they are trying to be overly responsible and/or they fail to set appropriate limits.

One therapist consistently felt overburdened by his patients. Many had chaotic lives and as they recited their litany of problems, he would think: "There is so much going wrong. This is too overwhelming. How am I ever going to make a dent with this patient?" On a practical level, the therapist needed to learn to help patients identify just one or two problems to focus on during each session. On a psychological level, the therapist needed to modify his overly responsible beliefs: "I should be able to help all my patients with all their problems. I should go the extra mile for all my patients, even when doing so is at significant cost to me." The therapist needed to change his expectations for himself, examine the limits and boundaries he set, and engage in better self-care.

When Therapists Believe They Will Displease Patients

Some therapists are concerned that their patients will get annoyed with them if they conduct therapy in a standard way (e.g., interrupt, structure the session, gently confront them).

Martha talked nearly nonstop. When her therapist tentatively attempted to get a word in edgewise, she ignored him. The therapist thought, "If I try harder to get her to stop, she'll get mad." The therapist was afraid that he would then not know what to do and the patient would terminate treatment. It was not until he consulted with a colleague that he recognized his own catastrophizing. He role-played how he could tactfully explain the need to interrupt and structure the session. He did a behavioral experiment and, to his surprise, found that the patient did not mind his directing the session. Had Martha become upset, though, he could have told her he was sorry she was distressed, discussed the problem directly with her, and negotiated a compromise.

When Therapists Feel Too Anxious about Patients

Therapists are understandably anxious when patients are at risk for hurting themselves or others. However, sometimes they unduly transmit their anxiety to the patient or their anxiety interferes with carrying out appropriate and effective therapy.

Doris had made three suicide attempts in the past 2 years and currently was intermittently suicidal. Her therapist was anxious, fearing that if he did not help the patient enough, Doris might make another attempt—this time, a lethal one. Doris sensed that her therapist was distressed, but she misperceived the nature of his distress. Instead of realizing that her therapist was anxious, she misperceived him as frustrated with her. Doris thought, "He thinks I can't be helped." This thought increased her sense of hopelessness and suicidal risk. Fortunately the therapist was able to elicit Doris's thinking and he acknowledged his fear that Doris might make another suicide attempt before he had a chance to really help her. Her therapist also consulted with colleagues, read up on dealing with suicidal patients, increased his frequency of contact with Doris, and had two family sessions. Once he felt more competent in dealing with Doris's suicidality, his anxiety decreased to a more manageable level.

When Therapists Feel Demeaned by Patients

Some patients who feel inferior develop a coping strategy of putting other people down. Therapists who have a propensity to feel inferior to others may feel disrespected and behave maladaptively toward these patients.

> Carly's therapist correctly perceived that his patient was demeaning of him from their very first session. She put him down whenever possible, tried to show off her intelligence, and mocked him when he did not know answers to her questions. The therapist's beliefs about his own inferiority became activated and he verbally disparaged the patient in their third session. Predictably, Carly walked out of the session and did not return to treatment. The therapist should have said to himself: "Carly is probably feeling inferior to me. She's reacting as if she's a vulnerable teenager who only knows how to flail out when she feels inferior. I should empathize with her and try to deactivate her inferiority belief." Had her therapist been able to conceptualize Carly accurately and respond to his own beliefs of inferiority, he might have fielded a challenge from her in a more functional way.

CARLY: You mean you don't think I had difficulty resolving the oral stage of psychosexual development! Don't you think you should know more about psychoanalytic theory? Shouldn't the PhD after your name *mean* something?

THERAPIST: Actually, you're probably right. I probably *should* know more about psychoanalytic theory. (*pause*) Are you concerned about that?

CARLY: Of course I am. I'm not sure you can really help me. Maybe I should see the director of the clinic, see what she says.

THERAPIST: (*nondefensively*) Sure. I'm sure she'd be willing to have a consultation with you, or with you and me, if you'd prefer. I always think two heads are better than one.

CARLY: (*Mutters.*) Well, I'll think about it.

THERAPIST: Okay. Now, for the time being, would you like to get back to talking about the incident with your mother?

When Therapists Feel Defensive

Often feelings of defensiveness arise when therapists feel criticized and blamed. Instead of viewing criticism and blame as a problem to be solved, they in turn blame the patient.

At their fifth session, Evelyn said in an annoyed tone, "You know, I think I should be feeling better by now. I've been coming here for, what, like 5 weeks—and I still feel the same. I don't think you know what you're doing." Her therapist thought: "I've been doing the right thing. It's *her* fault—she won't do the homework." Aloud he said, "Well, I'm not sure that's true. I think that if you had followed through with the assignments between sessions, you'd be feeling better now." The patient naturally felt blamed and the therapeutic relationship deteriorated further. A more adaptive exchange would have started with an empathic response, followed by collaborative problem solving:

THERAPIST: I'm sorry you're not feeling better. It must be really frustrating for you.

EVELYN: It is!

THERAPIST: Can you tell me what you think we've been doing wrong—and how you think therapy should go?

Such an exchange often disarms the patient and can lead to a more effective treatment plan.

When Therapists Feel Frustrated or Angry with Patients

Frustration or anger often arises when therapists have unrealistic expectations for their patients:

- "My patient should be cooperative/appreciative/easy to help/an active participant in therapy."
- "He shouldn't be difficult/manipulative/demanding."

In fact, it is helpful to recognize that patients *should* be exactly how they are, given their genetic predisposition, experiences, beliefs, and strategies. Therapists need to increase their empathy when they are frustrated or angry, recognizing that they themselves need to change their attitudes (and sometimes their general strategy and behavior) if patients are to progress.

Rodney's therapist became annoyed with him for trying to manipulate her into prescribing anxiolytic medication, when the patient had abused such medication in the past. Her thoughts were: "He shouldn't be asking me for meds. He's trying to make me feel sorry for him and manipulate me so I'll just give him the drugs. He's breaking our agreement." A more adaptive view would have been: "This was predictable. Of course he's going to seek drugs. He doesn't think he can feel better any other way. I don't have to argue with him, though. I can just firmly state the limit." With this view, the therapist is able to empathize with the patient and follow through more adaptively:

THERAPIST: I'm sorry you're feeling so bad—and you've probably already figured out that I have to turn you down, since [this medication] has been a problem for you in the past. (*pause*) What I can do, though, is to help you figure out how you can feel better without this kind of medication. (*pause*) Okay?

Therapists often get angry at patients who get angry at them.

Sharon became quite annoyed when her therapist again set a limit on between-session phone calls with her. The patient had responded quite angrily: "You don't understand. I don't call you all the time, only when I'm so upset I can't stand it! You don't care about me. You treat me like everyone else. I'm just another case to you." The therapist's automatic thoughts were: "Sharon is a pain in the neck. She overreacts all the time. Doesn't she realize I have to have a life myself!" A more adaptive view would have been empathic: "Poor Sharon. She has such a low threshold for tolerating feeling badly. It must be really hard for her." Such a view would have then led to a more adaptive response, starting with empathy:

THERAPIST: I'm really sorry I can't be there for you all the time. In some ways, it would be wonderful if you could reach me any time, day or night— and get immediate help. (*pause*) Of course, getting a quick fix has its downsides, too. You'd probably think you couldn't get along without me, and that would probably be pretty scary. (*pause*) So how about if we see if we can solve this problem together in another way. Are you willing?

When Therapists Feel Threatened by Patients

It should be noted that there are limits to what therapists should endure. Specifically, when therapists have good reason to believe that they (or their families) are at risk for harm as a result of a patient's behavior, they may ethically choose to discontinue their association with the patient (see Thompson, 1990). While it is true that therapists bear the major part of the burden of behaving in a mature, responsible manner in handling the difficulties of a strained therapeutic alliance, it is also true that they have a right to self-preservation. In cases where patients pose a real hazard to their therapists, the latter's responsibility to themselves, their families, and their other patients supersedes the need to "fix" the problem with the dangerous patient at all costs.

When Patients Bring Up a Therapist Reaction Problem

Occasionally, patients themselves bring up a therapist reaction problem, stating how they perceive their therapist is feeling. They may accurately perceive that their therapist is uncomfortable or distressed but draw an inaccurate conclusion. Therapists need to correct the misunderstanding honestly.

PATIENT: You must be getting so frustrated with me.

THERAPIST: What makes you think that?

PATIENT: I don't know. You seem . . . edgy or something.

THERAPIST: Well, I'm glad you told me. No, I'm not feeling frustrated. (*Thinks.*) But I think I am feeling a little anxious. I really want to help you with [this problem].

Sometimes patients *accurately* perceive their therapist's negative reaction. Therapists need to be as honestly positive as they can be, as was illustrated in the previous chapter. A good response to patients who are actually quite challenging is the following:

PATIENT: You think I'm a pain in the neck.

THERAPIST: Why do you say that?

PATIENT: I know I'm not an easy patient.

THERAPIST: That's for sure; you're not. To be honest, you can really be a challenge. But I like challenges. You always keep me thinking.

SUMMARY

Because therapists are human, it is inevitable, and sometimes even helpful, that they occasionally have a dysfunctional reaction toward their patients. As professionals, therapists need to conceptualize why the problem arose so they can take stock of their contribution to the problem and solve it. Working through the problem can be an important growth experience for therapists as they learn to modify their own thinking and behavior and broaden their repertoire for effectively managing patients with difficult problems. Consultations or ongoing supervision can be invaluable—and essential, in some cases—in order to assess and change a dysfunctional pattern, and to maximize the chances that the therapist will be able to respond in a more helpful, hopeful way in the future.

CHAPTER 7

Challenges in Setting Goals

Patients must have a clear idea of what they are working toward in therapy in order to keep their treatment on track and improve their motivation. Therapists generally start a goal list with patients in the first therapy session and add to it when additional problems or objectives are identified in future sessions. It is useful to review the goal list periodically and to ask patients how important each goal still is to them. Doing so helps remind patients that they are in therapy not to please the therapist and not simply to describe problems but instead to accomplish what is important to *them*. Goal lists are actually the flip side of problem lists, stated in a specific, behavioral way that implies solutions. Changing a problem of "loneliness," for example, to "Meet new people" and "Make plans with friends," specifies concrete goals that the patient can work toward achieving.

This chapter focuses on *setting* goals; working toward *achieving* goals is covered in Chapter 8, which focuses on solving problems and changing behavior. As with most therapeutic problems, there may be a practical problem (e.g., the therapist does not ask the patient to specify a general goal), a psychological problem (e.g., the patient has interfering beliefs such as "If I set goals, I'll have to do things I don't want to do") or both.

Employing and varying standard strategies to set goals is described first in this chapter. Typical dysfunctional beliefs and behaviors that interfere with goal setting are presented next. Finally, strategies to modify—or work around—dysfunctional beliefs that impede goal setting are provided and illustrated with case examples.

USING AND VARYING STANDARD STRATEGIES TO SET GOALS

Some problems arise in setting goals not because patients are resistant, but because therapists are not employing standard techniques effectively. For example, therapists may set goals with patients that are too broad, they may not address patients' hopelessness adequately, or they may not help patients change goals for other people into goals for themselves.

Setting Specific Goals through Questioning

When therapists ask patients about their goals for therapy, patients invariably reply with a broad, general goal: "I'd like to be happier" or "I don't want to be anxious any more." It is quite difficult for therapists to know precisely how to achieve such broad goals. A typical error therapists make is not questioning further to help patients *specify* their goals:

> ■ "How would you like to be different—or like your life to be different—as a result of therapy?"
> ■ "What changes would you like to make [in work, relationships, household management, your physical health, your spiritual/cultural/intellectual side]?"
> ■ "What would your life look like if you were happier?"

Therapists can also use pie charts to help patients compare how much time they currently spend in various activities versus how they would ideally like to spend their time. This procedure can also lead to specific goals patients would like to accomplish (J. Beck, 1995). Identification of specific goals that patients can work toward week by week facilitates therapy; failure to do so can impede therapy, as illustrated below.

Case Example

Jessica, a patient with bipolar disorder, set just one goal: to be happier. She did not see a connection between this broad goal and specific behavioral changes she needed to make, so she subsequently resisted her therapist's attempts to get her to regulate her life better by planning her days, completing projects, and normalizing her eating, sleeping, and activity levels. In fact, she saw these behaviors as interfering with potential happiness because she perceived them as inhibiting spontaneity and fun. It was not until her therapist asked her what her life would look like if she were happier that Jessica put her long-term goals into words: she wanted to be in a stable, intimate relationship; to get along better with her family; to succeed in a job that would nurture her artistic skills; and to save money to buy a car. After specifying her goals, Jessica became more willing to work on the immediate steps she needed to take to achieve them.

Setting Specific Goals through Imagery

Imaginal techniques can help patients who have difficulty setting goals. Therapists help patients picture in their minds a typical day that they hope to experience in the future. They ask leading questions so patients can picture themselves behaving functionally and feeling well.

> ■ "Can you imagine that it is a year from now and you're feeling significantly better? Let's talk about what your life looks like. Let's say it's a weekday morning. You're feeling better, you've slept well, you have some energy. What time do you get up in the morning? Can you picture yourself getting out of bed? How are you feeling? What do you do next? Do you get right out of bed? Go right to the kitchen and turn the coffee on? *What do you want to imagine you do next?* Next? . . . Next?"

Therapists continue to question patients, encouraging them to visualize such scenes in their minds. They may need to use additional leading questions:

> ■ "Okay, it's lunchtime. What do you want to imagine happens next? Do you see yourself asking [your coworker] Joan to have lunch with you? Can you see yourself walking to lunch? Describe it to me . . . . How are you feeling? . . . . What do you talk about at lunch?. . . . What do you want to imagine you do next?"

It is helpful to continue the image until patients see themselves in bed for the night, drifting off to sleep, contemplating the satisfying day they have had. Following this imagery exercise, the therapist and the patient can discuss the differences between this desired scenario and what the patient is currently doing in order to set specific goals.

Imagery can be used in another way, too. When patients are too hopeless about their future to envision a better day to come, their therapists can ask them to imagine and describe a typical day in the past when they remember feeling well. They then help patients identify specific differences between their behavior at that time and their current behavior in order to identify changes the patient might need to make.

Case Example

Allen was feeling so hopeless that he did not respond to the standard goal-setting questions and had difficulty imagining a future scene.

THERAPIST: Is it okay if we talk about your goals for therapy now?

ALLEN: (*Sighs.*) I guess.

THERAPIST: How would you like to be different as a result of therapy? How would you like your life to be different?

ALLEN: (*in a low voice*) I don't know. I don't know what being undepressed would be like any more. Feels like I've been [depressed] like this forever.

THERAPIST: (*asking a leading question*) I wonder, could you imagine what your day might be like, say, a year from now, if you were back to your old self, feeling pretty good, not depressed, but pretty energetic, motivated, and so on? (*getting specific*) What time would you get out of bed, for example?

ALLEN: I don't know. I can't imagine *not* feeling like this.

THERAPIST: You're feeling pretty down.

ALLEN: Yeah.

THERAPIST: I wonder, could you tell me instead about the last time you did feel like your old self? When would that have been?

ALLEN: (*Thinks.*) Oh, boy. (*Sighs.*) That was a long time ago.

THERAPIST: Was it when you were still working at [a local company]?

ALLEN: (*Thinks.*) Yeah, I guess so.

THERAPIST: Can you tell me a little about what your life was like then? How you were feeling?

ALLEN: I was feeling pretty good, I think. I liked my job. I was really into playing basketball with some friends . . . .

THERAPIST: What was your energy level like?

ALLEN: Good. No problem.

THERAPIST: What did you like about your job?

The therapist engaged the patient, getting him to recall a better time in his life. She helped Allen create a vision and collected data by asking questions about his activities, mood, relationships, and view of himself. As she helped him set goals by identifying activities and behaviors he was no longer engaged in, she also had to help Allen with his interfering automatic thoughts, do some problem solving, and suggest alternate ways of viewing the situation.

THERAPIST: So what do you think of the idea of starting running again?

ALLEN: I don't know. It would take a really long time to get back in shape. I used to be able to run 2, 3 miles a day.

THERAPIST: So what do you think? Would it be better not to run at all? Or maybe to have a goal to start off small and build up your endurance a little bit each week?

ALLEN: I guess.

THERAPIST: Okay, could you write that down? And I guess it will be important to give yourself credit when you run, even if it's only for two blocks. (*pause*) I assume two blocks is better than no blocks?

ALLEN: Yeah.

THERAPIST: Okay, that sounds good. (*pause*) Now, you also mentioned that you used to hang out at your sister's house sometimes, play with her kids, help her out. (*pause*) Is that something that would be good for you to start doing again?

ALLEN: (*Looks downcast.*) Maybe. But her kids are older now. I'm not sure they'd want to hang out with me.

THERAPIST: Well, you might be right about that. Or you might just have to change what you do with them. (*offering a forced choice*) Which kid do you think might be most receptive?

ALLEN: (*Thinks.*) The youngest, Joey.

THERAPIST: How old is he now?

ALLEN: I don't know. Eight, 9?

THERAPIST: What could you do with him? (*pause*) What did *you* used to like to do when you were 8 or 9?

The therapist continues to help the patient set goals, based on the memories he has of his "old self," creatively working around his hopelessness.

Changing Goals Set for Others to Personal Goals

Patients sometimes set goals for other people instead of for themselves: "I want my boss to stop pressuring me"; "I want my husband to stop drinking"; "I want my kids to listen to me." If patients do not have interfering dysfunctional beliefs (such as "If I set goals for myself, I'll have to be responsible for changing" or "It isn't fair that I have to change"), it is relatively easy to help them understand that they and their therapist, working together, can not directly change the other person. They are usually willing to accept a goal that is under their own control.

THERAPIST: How do you want your life to be as a result of therapy? What do you want to do differently?

PATIENT: I want my wife to appreciate me more. She's always nagging me, do this, do that. I can't understand why she doesn't understand *how much I do for her*! You know, I really go out of my way to make her happy. I work hard, I don't run around [with other women], I bring home my paycheck every week.

THERAPIST: (*empathically*) Sounds pretty frustrating. (*pause*) It sounds like it would be a good goal to improve things with your wife. (*pause*) But I don't want to mislead you and tell you that our therapy can *directly* change her—not unless you think she'd be willing to come in for therapy and set that goal for herself?

PATIENT: (*glumly*) No, she wouldn't.

THERAPIST: Then maybe we should see what goal we could set that *you* have control over. (*pause*) What have you been doing up to this point to try to get her to appreciate you?

PATIENT: (*Thinks.*) Every time I hand her my paycheck to deposit, I remind her that I'm working hard for the family.

THERAPIST: Anything else?

PATIENT: (*Shrugs.*)

THERAPIST: Do you *tell* her she should appreciate you more?

PATIENT: Well, sure. Especially when she's on my back for not doing something.

THERAPIST: How well are those things working to get her appreciation?

PATIENT: (*sourly*) They're not.

THERAPIST: Do you think if you keep on doing these things she's likely to suddenly change and become appreciative?

PATIENT: (*Thinks.*) No, probably not.

THERAPIST: So, one goal for therapy could be to learn what *you* can do differently, what other things *you* might be able to say to your wife. (*pause*) Maybe then she'd respond differently to you. (*pause*) What do you think?

PATIENT: I suppose.

THERAPIST: Okay, so one goal might be "Learn different ways to talk to wife." Is that okay?

PATIENT: Yeah.

PATIENTS' DYSFUNCTIONAL BELIEFS ABOUT SETTING GOALS

A certain percentage of patients do not respond well to the standard techniques described above. Often they hold dysfunctional beliefs about themselves, about others, or about the therapist. When therapists ask such patients about the goals they would like to achieve, their core beliefs may become activated: "I'm helpless," "I'm incompetent," "I'm vulnerable," "I'm worthless." Patients may make certain assumptions about the outcome or meaning of setting goals, changing, and/or getting better. These assumptions are, in turn, associated with the dysfunctional behavior they display in session.

Assumptions about Themselves

"If I set goals, I'll feel bad (e.g., I'll be overwhelmed by all the things I have to do)."

"If I set goals, I'll have to change."

"If I have to change, it means I've been wrong or bad."

"If I try to change, I'll fail."

"If I change, it will invalidate my suffering."

"If I change, my life will get worse."

"I don't deserve to change and have a better life."

"It's not fair that I have to change."

Assumptions about Others

"If I change, it will let other people (who should be punished) off the hook."

"If I change, other people will expect more and more from me."

Assumptions about the Therapist

"If I set goals (as my therapist requests), it means she's in control and I'm weak."

"If I set goals, I'll have to reveal myself to the therapist (and I could get hurt)."

DYSFUNCTIONAL BEHAVIORS

When patients hold the kinds of assumptions listed above, they may display behaviors such as the following:

- Denying that problems exist (so setting goals is not relevant).
- Blaming problems on others and setting goals for others.
- Declaring that therapy cannot help (so it is useless to set goals).
- Stating that they are too helpless or inadequate to change.
- Setting unrealistic goals.
- Setting goals related only to an existential search for meaning.

THERAPEUTIC STRATEGIES

A number of strategies can be helpful when patients resist setting goals or set unhelpful goals due to their dysfunctional beliefs:

- Eliciting and responding to automatic thoughts that interfere with goal setting.
- Acknowledging to skeptical patients that therapy is not guaranteed to be successful but that the therapist is hopeful, based on what he/she knows thus far about the patient.
- Helping patients see that continuing to live, act, and think the way they currently do will likely make them feel worse, not better.
- Helping patients understand which goals they have control over and which they do not; helping patients turn goals they have set for other people into goals they themselves can accomplish.
- Turning patients' complaints and dissatisfactions into goals.
- Educating biologically oriented patients about how therapy can help reduce physiological symptoms.
- Delaying setting existential goals until the patient is less symptomatic.
- Letting patients have more control in the session when pushing to set goals is damaging the therapeutic alliance (e.g., initially accepting broad or vague goals, identifying just one goal, or delaying formal goal setting).

These strategies are illustrated in the case examples below.

Case Example 1: The Patient Who Feels Too Hopeless to Set Goals

Thomas was a 32-year-old man with recurrent severe depression. He had just been fired from yet another job, his family had distanced themselves from him and he had no close friends or intimate relationships. In addition, he was experiencing uncomfortable side effects from his medication, which he took sporadically. Initially he was nonresponsive to his therapist's efforts to set goals.

THERAPIST: Thomas, what are your goals for therapy?

THOMAS: (*Looks down.*) I don't know.

THERAPIST: How would you like to be different as a result of therapy?

THOMAS: (*Mumbles.*) I don't know.

THERAPIST: It doesn't sound as if things are going too well for you right now.

THOMAS: (*mumbling, looking down*) No.

THERAPIST: And they haven't for a while?

THOMAS: No.

THERAPIST: If there was one thing about your life you could change, what would it be?

THOMAS: I don't know.

THERAPIST: (*pause*) And how are you feeling right now?

THOMAS: (*Looks down.*)

THERAPIST: Not too good?

THOMAS: No.

THERAPIST: Sad? Worried? Hopeless?

THOMAS: (*Thinks.*) Down. Real down.

THERAPIST: (*hypothesizing about his automatic thoughts*) Are you thinking therapy won't help?

THOMAS: (*pauses*) Yeah.

THERAPIST: Because it's not the right kind of therapy? Because I'm not the right kind of therapist?

THOMAS: (*Thinks.*) No.

THERAPIST: Is it something about *you*?

THOMAS: (*softly, still looking down*) Yeah.

THERAPIST: Are you feeling kind of helpless?

THOMAS: (*Nods.*)

THERAPIST: Like there's nothing you can do?

THOMAS: Yeah.

THERAPIST: How much do you believe that thought, that there's nothing you can do?

THOMAS: (*pauses*) A lot.

THERAPIST: You feel kind of stuck?

THOMAS: Yeah.

THERAPIST: Well, would you be willing to let me help you figure out whether you can get unstuck?

THOMAS: (*pauses*) I don't think I can.

THERAPIST: Well you might be right about that . . . or you might be wrong. Nearly every depressed patient who walks through that door for the first time feels pretty hopeless . . . . But I do have a pretty good track record of helping people.

THOMAS: Hmmm.

THERAPIST: One thing I know, though, is that it's hard to get going when you don't know what you're aiming for. . . . For example, would you like to find a job that you can keep? Do you want to get more involved with people?

THOMAS: (*still looking down*) I don't know.

THERAPIST: (*collecting more information*) What would be the downside?

THOMAS: I just don't think it will happen. I've been struggling and struggling for a long time. Nothing has worked out.

THERAPIST: (*hypothesizing*) Are you afraid of getting your hopes up?

THOMAS: (*Nods.*)

THERAPIST: (*normalizing his reaction*) Well, I guess if I were in your shoes, I might not want to get my hopes up either. . . . All I can say is there's *nothing about you* that makes me think this therapy *won't* work. . . . Would you be willing to work with me for at least four sessions—and then we can decide together if it's helping or not?

THOMAS: (*Nods.*)

THERAPIST: So could we talk about what might be reasonable to try to accomplish in the next 4 weeks?

THOMAS: Okay.

THERAPIST: I see from this paper you filled out [describing his current functioning] that you're having trouble organizing things at home. Can you tell me a little about that?

They then discuss small goals related to cleaning up at home (e.g., throwing away trash, collecting all the bills in one place, cleaning up the kitchen). The therapist also ascertains that the patient does not know about social services for which he might be eligible, so they set a goal for him to call and ask for information. Other goals included calling a cousin, seeing his psychiatrist for a medication check, and going bowling.

Why was goal setting so difficult for Thomas? In the next few sessions, his therapist confirmed her hypotheses about him. Thomas had a core belief that he was incapable and a failure; he assumed that no matter what he tried, he would fail. The strategy he demonstrated in therapy was avoidance: he avoided any activity that he predicted would result in failure. And because he felt vulnerable to falling into the depths of depression, he avoided feeling hopeful. (See Moore & Garland, 2003, for more on addressing hopelessness in chronically depressed patients.)

Case Example 2: The Patient Who Refuses to Define Her Goals

Erica, a 57-year-old woman, was divorced, on disability, and spent most of her time housebound, caring for her verbally abusive mother. Erica had had a horrible childhood in which she endured significant emotional, physical, and sexual abuse. She had a long history of hospitalizations for suicide attempts, of partial hospitalizations, and outpatient group and individual therapy. In the first session, her new therapist tried to set goals.

THERAPIST: Erica, what are your goals for therapy? How do you want to be different as a result of therapy?

ERICA: (*long pause, speaks almost inaudibly*) I don't want to be in this much pain.

THERAPIST: (*softly*) Of course. That's so important. (*pause*) If your pain were *reduced* (*not wanting to sound overly optimistic*), what would your life look like? How might it be different?

ERICA: (*long pause*) It wouldn't, I guess.

THERAPIST: So you'd be doing the same things, but feel less pain?

ERICA: (*pause*) I guess so.

THERAPIST: Is there anything about your life you'd *like* to change? (*realizing that providing a multiple-choice question may be easier for the patient to respond to than an open-ended question*) Be more involved with people? Get back to work? (*pause*) Put some enjoyment in your life?

ERICA: (*Sighs, pauses.*) No, I don't think so.

THERAPIST: Because?

ERICA: (*a little irritably*) It's not going to happen.

THERAPIST: You don't think you can change?

ERICA: (*irritably*) No.

THERAPIST: Okay, for now then, how about if we just work toward reducing your pain.

ERICA: (*Nods.*)

The therapist sensed that continuing to talk about goals at this time would alienate Erica. They had a tenuous alliance at best and the therapist's overriding goal in this first session was to create an atmosphere that the patient perceived as safe enough to be willing to return for the next session.

Erica did return the following week and provided data that helped the therapist conceptualize why they had had difficulty setting goals in the previous session. In the context of activity scheduling, the patient revealed that she saw herself as bad and undeserving of pleasure. In fact, she believed that she deserved to be *punished* if she did things to make herself feel better. Her strategy in session was to resist attempts (including goal setting) to feel better. In fact, the therapist was not able to get her to set goals until several things occurred in therapy:

- The therapist changed her question from how Erica would like to be different as a result of therapy to "What do you think you *should* be doing differently?"
- The patient trusted the therapist more (no longer believing that the therapist would try to force her to do things she felt uncomfortable doing—especially pleasurable activities).
- The patient started to modify her core belief about being bad and her assumption that she deserved punishment for feeling pleasure. (See Chapters 12 and 13.)

Case Example 3: The Patient Who Denies She Has a Problem

Lisa was a 15-year-old girl with mild depression who showed signs of oppositional–defiance disorder. Her mother had insisted she come to therapy. The mother reported that Lisa had grown increasingly uncooperative at home. She was moody and fought constantly with her mom and younger brothers. Lisa was failing several subjects at school and her mother suspected she was using drugs. Lisa made it clear from the beginning that she was an unwilling participant in therapy.

THERAPIST: Lisa, would it be okay if we talked about what you want to get out of therapy?

LISA: (*Shrugs.*)

THERAPIST: How would you like to be different—or how would you like your life to be different?

LISA: I don't even know why I'm here. I told you before, it's my mother who needs therapy. She's really psycho. Ever since my dad left—which, by the way, was *totally her fault*, she's been getting worse and worse. You ask anyone—my brothers, my Aunt Flo, everyone will tell you how out of control she is.

THERAPIST: (*mildly*) I guess she sees it differently?

LISA: (*angrily*) She thinks *I* have a problem. (*sarcastically*) That's really funny.

THERAPIST: (*empathically*) Sounds like you're really stuck. Here *she's* the one with the problem but she's making *you* come to therapy.

LISA: (*Mutters.*) Everything would be fine, just fine, if I didn't have to deal with her.

THERAPIST: (*collecting data*) Any chance of that happening?

LISA: No. Not for a long time, anyway.

THERAPIST: So you're stuck dealing with her.

LISA: Yeah.

THERAPIST: Can you give me some idea of what it's like, trying to deal with her?

LISA: (*speaking in general terms*) She's impossible.

THERAPIST: (*trying to get the Lisa to be more specific*) What bothers you the most?

LISA: Oh, everything. I don't even want to *look* at her any more.

THERAPIST: (*empathically*) Things are that bad?

LISA: Yeah.

THERAPIST: Well, I would like to see if there's something you and I could do to improve things for you.

LISA: (*Looks at the ceiling.*)

THERAPIST: I gather from your silence that you don't like that idea?

LISA: It's not *fair* that *I* should have to improve things when *she's* the problem. I just want her to get off my back. (*in an accusing tone*) But you're probably going to tell me that I need to be (*in a sarcastic tone*) *polite* to my mom and *cooperate* and be a *good daughter*.

THERAPIST: Uh, oh. I'm glad you told me that. Okay, I will try *not* to say those things. But, Lisa, I might slip. And if I do, I'm going to need you to catch me so I can correct myself. (*pause*) Would you be willing to do that?

LISA: (*surprised*) Yeah, yeah, I will.

THERAPIST: Good, because if you don't, I don't think this therapy is going to work.

Here the therapist recognized that they would have to deal with a therapeutic relationship problem before the patient would be willing to set goals. The therapist purposely tried to redress the balance of power in their relationship by agreeing to what the patient wanted, and, in fact, asking the patient to correct her when she makes a mistake. Then they return to goal setting.

THERAPIST: So, back to what you want to get out of therapy.

LISA: (*setting a goal for another person*) Make my mom be nice to me.

THERAPIST: Do you think that's something *you* can make happen?

LISA: (*glumly*) No.

THERAPIST: So, it's not something you have *direct* control over (*implying she may have indirect control*).

LISA: No, but maybe *you* could talk to her.

THERAPIST: Yeah, I definitely want for *both of us* to talk to her together.

Remember I told you I want to call her in here toward the end of the session?

LISA: (*Nods.*)

THERAPIST: Meanwhile, can we talk about what you *do* have control over?

LISA: (*Thinks for a while.*) I don't know. It's so awful. From the time she gets home from work till the time she goes to sleep, she's fighting with me and my brothers. Constantly. It's like there's no place I can go and just be quiet.

THERAPIST: (*empathically*) That *is* terrible. (*using self-disclosure*) Like when I've worked all day and go home, I know sometime during the evening I'm going to be able to just sit down and relax. (*pause*) It doesn't sound like it's that way for you.

LISA: No. My mom is always on me. As soon as I walk in the door, she's on me. "Do this, do that." I mean, before I've even taken off my coat. And then she hates it when I'm just sitting watching TV. She gets all sarcastic and makes me turn it off. And my brothers—they're so annoying, too.

THERAPIST: Boy, you really *do* need some quiet time at home . . . . Should we make that a goal?

LISA: Yeah.

Here the therapist seized on a complaint and turned it into a specific goal that the patient agrees with.

THERAPIST: Do you think your mom would agree?

LISA: No. She'd probably say that I can't have quiet time till I've finished all the stuff she wants me to do. Plus she'll say homework comes first. She's so impossible.

THERAPIST: So maybe we should figure out now what both of us could say to her.

LISA: Okay.

What were Lisa's initial beliefs and strategies that made it difficult for her to set goals? First, she had core beliefs that she was helpless and that others, especially her mother, controlled her. She made several dysfunctional assumptions:

"If I try to change my life, I won't be able to."
"If I acknowledge that I play a part in my difficulties, I'll have to take responsibility for changing."

"If I change, Mom wins."

"If I change, I won't be able to punish Mom."

"If I do as my therapist says, it means she's in control and I'm not."

So the strategy Lisa used in session was to blame her mother for all her problems and initially to resist setting goals for herself. Rather than continuing to try to set goals in this first session, the therapist decides that making some headway on Lisa's desire to gain quiet time will strengthen the therapeutic alliance and make Lisa more amenable to goal setting in the next session. Therefore they formulate a reasonable schedule that Lisa thinks she could get her mother to agree to and they role-play what Lisa can say to her mom when her mother joins them toward the end of the therapy session. The therapist helps Lisa see that this new way of talking to her mother, even if it is polite and cooperative, is designed to help Lisa be more in control of the relationship with her mother and to get what Lisa wants.

Experiencing even some limited success at home in gaining quiet time influenced Lisa's attitude toward therapy. She began to believe that perhaps therapy might help and that she could gain more control in making her life better. Indeed, Lisa was at least minimally more amenable in the next few therapy sessions to discussing her long-term goals and the steps she needed to start taking in the short run.

Case Example 4: The Patient Who Believes His Problems Are Entirely Physical

Greg was a 32-year-old unmarried carpenter who entered treatment for panic disorder. He was sure that the problem was not psychological, however, and came to therapy only because his cardiologist had insisted. Greg had had extensive medical workups and tests and had visited the emergency room four times in the previous 6 weeks. In the first session, the therapist started to set goals, then found that she needed to do some psychoeducation.

THERAPIST: I'd like to talk to you a little bit now about goals for therapy. I assume the major one is to get over your panic disorder?

GREG: Yeah . . . but to tell the truth, I don't know that you can help me there.

THERAPIST: You don't think therapy can help you get over this? Or that *I* can't.

GREG: No, no, it's not you, doc. But to be honest, I'm only here because my doctor insisted I come.

THERAPIST: Do you know why he wanted you to come here?

GREG: Well, he said this therapy would help. But, see, I don't really think so. I mean, obviously there's something wrong with me. Talking can't help that.

THERAPIST: (*clarifying*) Something wrong with you *physically*.

GREG: Yeah.

THERAPIST: Well, you're right. Obviously there *is* something wrong with you physically. From what you say, your heart speeds up and starts to pound, your chest gets all tight, you have trouble getting your breath. Of course it's physical.

GREG: Then why ... ?

THERAPIST: Why do I think I can help you?

GREG: (*Nods.*)

The therapist then discusses the cognitive model of panic and an evolutionary explanation for an overactive built-in alarm system in the brain (Clark & Ehlers, 1993). The patient is still skeptical.

THERAPIST: Well, I guess there are two possibilities. One is that you really *are* in danger when you get those terrible sensations .... *Or*, as I was saying before, you're *not* in danger of having a heart attack but your body keeps getting more and more revved up because you are *convinced* that you're having a heart attack.

GREG: Yeah.

THERAPIST: So, as I see it, you have two choices. You can *assume* that there is something life-threateningly wrong with you that the doctors haven't found yet and keep going the medical route—though you told me your doctor said they had run every test they could and the emergency room docs never found anything wrong with your heart.

GREG: (*Nods.*)

THERAPIST: Or you can come back next week (*implying that the patient doesn't have to make a longer commitment*) and together we can try to figure out whether you need a purely medical approach or whether a cognitive therapy approach might help. (*pause*) What do you think?

Greg's core belief was that he was vulnerable. His assumption was that if he agreed to therapy instead of pursuing a medical route further, he would be harmed. So the strategy he uses in session is to insist that the problem is purely physical and to resist entertaining alternative explanations for his symptoms. The therapist provides additional psychoeducation and then offers the goal of a collaborative exploration to find the best treatment approach. Greg accepts this goal, albeit reluctantly, when his therapist suggests that he try cognitive therapy for just a limited number of sessions.

Case Example 5: The Patient Who Sets Unrealistic Goals

Stephanie is a 40-year-old married woman with two elementary school-age children. She is depressed and quite overwhelmed. She has full responsibility for raising the children and running the household. She also works full time in the bakery section of a supermarket. Her husband, Gene, is an auto mechanic at a local gas station. Stephanie recently started an affair with her married neighbor, Hal. Hal is 15 years younger than Stephanie and clearly seems interested only in a temporary sexual relationship.

THERAPIST: What do you want to get out of therapy? How do you want to be different?

STEPHANIE: I want Hal to spend more time with me. I want Gene to let me get a divorce, at least I think I do. I know he doesn't want that. He says he still loves me. I don't know how he could—after finding out about Hal, I mean. I don't want to hurt Gene. I wish he could just see that we have to go our separate ways. He isn't a bad husband. He should have someone who's really *in* love with him. I mean, I still love Gene, to a certain degree. I just don't want to be married to him any more. And I don't want the kids to be hurt. Already they're upset that I'm not home as much. They've gotten really clingy. I'm afraid Gene is going to give me a hard time about custody.

THERAPIST: (*jotting down goals*) Okay, let me make sure I got this right and that it's really under your control to accomplish these goals. One, you want Hal to spend more time with you. Two, you want, or you think you want, to get divorced and to do that without hurting Gene. Three, you don't want the kids to be hurt. Did I get that right?

STEPHANIE: Yeah.

THERAPIST: You know, Stephanie, I don't want to mislead you. I'm not sure it's under our control to make these things happen.

STEPHANIE: (*in a disappointed voice*) Oh.

THERAPIST: (*anticipating her automatic thought*) Which *doesn't* mean I can't help you—you're obviously depressed and anxious and you *need* help—but we may need to change the goals.

STEPHANIE: Do you think Hal will leave his wife for me?

THERAPIST: To be honest, I don't know enough about your relationship with him yet, but it doesn't sound good. Maybe that could be a goal: find out what Hal's intentions are. (*pause*) What do you think?

STEPHANIE: No. (*Thinks*) I'm afraid to. I don't want to push him. I think he'll drop me if I start talking to him about it.

THERAPIST: Doesn't sound like you have much control there.

STEPHANIE: No, he's really the one who decides stuff—like when we're going to get together.

THERAPIST: So this goal of having Hal spend more time with you—it might not be something *you* can decide to do, not if he's the one who's calling the shots.

Next, through the therapist's use of Socratic questioning, Stephanie concluded that it was unrealistic to expect that Gene would not be hurt by her seeing Hal and by discussing the possibility of divorce with him. The therapist also helped Stephanie see that her children were likely to continue to be upset, possibly becoming more so, if Stephanie continued to spend time with Hal instead of with them and if the arguments and constant tension between Stephanie and Gene continued.

THERAPIST: (*giving Stephanie permission to express her distress*) You know, if I were you, Stephanie, I'd be really disappointed by this discussion.

STEPHANIE: Yeah. I mean I know what you're saying, but I just can't face the idea of life without Hal.

THERAPIST: Oh. Let me think for a moment. I really do want to help you— I hope you know that. I'm just afraid of giving you false hope. . . . Okay, here's what I think. You told me that the only times you feel good nowadays are when you're with Hal or when you're thinking about being with him. Is that right?

STEPHANIE: (*Nods.*)

THERAPIST: On the other hand, we don't know that he wants a future with you the way you do with him. In fact, it *sounds* as if he doesn't— making plans with his wife to have another baby.

STEPHANIE: (*Makes a wry face.*)

THERAPIST: It seems to me that we have to figure out how you can feel good in other ways, too. So if Hal *does* break off the relationship with you, you'll still be able to have a good life. (*pause*) What do you think?

STEPHANIE: (*half-heartedly*) I suppose so. I don't know what else I could feel good about, though.

THERAPIST: Well, could that be a goal we work on together? Finding ways for you to feel good?

STEPHANIE: Yeah, I guess so.

THERAPIST: And now Gene. Sounds like part of you wants to divorce him, but part of you isn't completely sure. Would the goal be to make that decision?

STEPHANIE: Yeah, I know, I keep putting it off. I just wish *Gene* would up and leave *me*. That would make it so much easier.

THERAPIST: In some ways, probably. (*pause*) But that makes me a little confused. Is the goal to decide on whether or not to get a divorce? Or have you already decided and the goal is to help you through it and try not to devastate Gene?

STEPHANIE: I guess I'm still not sure.

THERAPIST: Okay, so the first goal is to decide. (*Writes that down.*) And, I guess, whatever the outcome, to try to reduce the arguing and tension with Gene?

STEPHANIE: Yeah.

At that point they discussed goals of dealing more effectively with the children, reducing the burdens of running the household, and planning more enjoyable activities that do not involve being with or fantasizing about Hal.

THERAPIST: (*having summarized the goal list*) How disappointed are you that the goals don't include making Hal want to spend more time with you? And getting divorced without hurting Gene and the kids?

STEPHANIE: (*Reflects.*) I *am* disappointed.

THERAPIST: So disappointed you won't want to come back next week?

STEPHANIE: No, I'll come back.

Here the therapist needed to help the patient set realistic goals. She had to be cognizant, though, that Stephanie might discontinue therapy if she confronted her too strongly. At the end, she gave the patient permission to express her disappointment with the therapist and ascertained her willingness to return to therapy.

Why did Stephanie have difficulty setting realistic goals? She had core beliefs of helplessness, vulnerability, and unlovability. Major dysfunctional assumptions included: "I can only be happy if I have Hal. If I stop seeing him and fantasizing about him, I'll feel terrible and won't be able to cope." A major coping strategy she used was to fantasize whenever she felt distressed and avoid thinking about problems.

Case Example 6: The Patient Who Sets Existential Goals

Arthur was a 31-year-old man suffering from major depression and early-onset chronic dysthymia on Axis I and avoidant personality disorder with strong narcissistic features on Axis II. He was unemployed, had never held a job for more than a year, had few friends, and was living with and was financially supported by his parents with whom he had a conflictual relationship. In the following part of the first session, Arthur laid out his existential concerns:

THERAPIST: So what are your goals for therapy?

ARTHUR: I have to tell you right off that I don't really have any. In fact, I don't know that therapy can help. I've been struggling for a long time. I've seen lots of therapists. (*pause*) But my life hasn't gotten any better. I just feel like it's so meaningless most of the time.

THERAPIST: So an important goal would be to help you find some meaning?

ARTHUR: Yeah. (*Sighs.*) But I'm not hopeful that'll happen.

THERAPIST: Well, let me ask you this. Can you picture a scenario in which you wake up and you think about your day and it automatically feels like you have a purpose—that you're going to do some things that are important?

ARTHUR: (*Thinks.*) No, I guess if I could do that I wouldn't have to come here.

THERAPIST: Do you have a sense of what other people have a sense of purpose about?

ARTHUR: Yeah, I guess so. . . . They have jobs they think are important, or families they have to provide for.

THERAPIST: Is that something you'd like to aim for?

ARTHUR: No, no, I don't think so.

THERAPIST: Because?

ARTHUR: I can't see myself feeling fulfilled in a job. Most work is boring. I know I'm not working now, but I've had a lot of jobs in the past. I've always hated them. I mean, what's the point? You slave away for a few bucks an hour while the boss or the owner of the company is making millions. Then you go home and pass the hours till you go to sleep and wake up and go to work again. And it's even worse if you have a wife and kids, or something, and have to keep working so they won't starve.

THERAPIST: Wow, that does sound bleak! No wonder you don't know if you can improve your life.

ARTHUR: What's it all for, anyway? You work, you eat, you sleep, and eventually you die.

The patient continued to describe his existential crisis for several minutes, questioning his place in the universe and the futility of working and trying to enjoy oneself, knowing that one will just die eventually. The therapist summarized the patient's concerns and confirmed that she had grasped his difficulties. Next, she provided some psychoeducation:

THERAPIST: You know, these are all important questions you have, essential questions. And I think therapy can help you figure out some of the answers, though many of us struggle with them to some degree throughout our lives. (*pause*) What we've found, though, is that people find these questions almost *impossible* to answer when they're depressed. (*pause*) Once they get treated for the depression and the depression lifts, then they have more success.

ARTHUR: Hmmm.

THERAPIST: What do you think about that?

ARTHUR: I don't know. (*pause*) I have to think about it. (*pause*) What would I have to do to get less depressed?

THERAPIST: (*anticipating Arthur will dismiss the plan*) Now, I'm not saying that the standard formula will work for you. But most people, with or without these kinds of questions, need to rearrange what they're doing. For example, you've told me that you spend most of your day watching television or reading the newspaper or going online. Is that formula working for you? Has it made you steadily less depressed?

ARTHUR: (*Thinks.*) No, I guess not.

THERAPIST: Then changing your activities is probably really important. And learning how to change your depressed thinking is also really important.

ARTHUR: I'm not sure I *want* to do that. I mean, I've tried that in the past and it's really never gotten me anyplace.

THERAPIST: And Arthur, I can't *guarantee* you that it will get you anyplace this time either. But tell me, in your previous therapy experiences, did you set specific goals like getting more satisfaction out of every day or learning what to do when you find you're thinking in a really depressed way? Did your therapists set agendas with you every session like I'm doing and give you some things to experiment with at home every week?

ARTHUR: No . . . .

THERAPIST: Well, that's good. Because if this therapy were exactly like your other experiences I would be less hopeful. (*anticipating that Arthur may be nervous about the changes he will have to make*) But let me tell you one other thing. It's hard for me to predict right now how quickly or slowly we'll need to go. If you've been stuck in this way of thinking and behaving for a long time, we may need to go more slowly. (*making Arthur feel more in control*) I'll need you to kind of set the pace. (*pause*) Would you be willing to think about this some more this week and come back next week to tell me whether you think this is the way to go—or whether we need to take another approach?

The therapist conceptualized that Arthur might be focused on existential questions as a strategy to avoid taking steps to move ahead in life (e.g., getting a job) because he predicted that he would meet with failure, as he had in the past. The therapist provided psychoeducation and the broad outlines of a tentative treatment plan and *avoided* asking Arthur to commit to therapy at this point. Instead she tried to get him to commit to returning the following week to work out a therapy plan that suits him. Arthur did return for a second session but was still uncertain about how therapy should proceed. The therapist engaged him in an examination of the advantages and disadvantages of focusing on existential questions initially versus the advantages and disadvantages of focusing on a more standard approach to treating his depression before they got to the existential issues.

Following this discussion, Arthur agreed to try the standard approach for 4 weeks, at which point he would assess whether he thought they were on the right track. Instead of setting comprehensive goals at this session, they set two relatively unthreatening goals: (1) Arthur would try to structure his time so that he could get more satisfaction and pleasure in what he did, and, (2) he would try to monitor and respond to depressing thoughts that interfered with his satisfaction and pleasure. The therapist postponed additional goal setting for several sessions until Arthur had had initial success with these goals and both she and the therapy had gained credibility in his eyes.

Arthur's core belief was that he was inadequate, inferior, and a failure. His assumption was that if he tried to improve his life, he would fail. Therefore he used a strategy of overly focusing on existential questions to avoid tackling today's problems.

Case Example 7: The Patient Who Avoids Setting an Important Goal

Jenna was a 19-year-old woman who lived with her parents. Her mother brought her to therapy for treatment of depression and anger. Jenna had abruptly quit her job as a waitress 3 weeks earlier, following a suicidal gesture, which was precipitated by a nasty rumor a coworker had spread about her. In this first session, Jenna anticipated that her therapist would try to make her return to the job and she put the therapist on notice that she had no intention of doing so.

THERAPIST: So what do you want to get out of therapy?

JENNA: (*in a sullen voice*) I don't know.

THERAPIST: Well, how would you like your life to be different?

JENNA: I know I'm supposed to say that I want to go back to my job but the truth is that I don't. (*forcefully*) And I *won't*. (*Looks menacingly at the therapist.*)

THERAPIST: I know the job was pretty bad for you last month.

JENNA: (*in a disgusted voice*) It sucks. The people who work there suck. The customers suck.

THERAPIST: Well, no wonder you don't want to go back.

JENNA: (*sarcastically*) Yeah, no kidding. Anyway, I *can't* go back. It's too upsetting. I'd probably get really depressed and just try to kill myself again.

THERAPIST: Well, I can see that I'd better not try to convince you to go back. What are your choices?

JENNA: I don't know. Stay home, I guess.

THERAPIST: Can you do that?

JENNA: My mother would kill me. She is so furious with me right now because I won't go to my job. She threatened to throw me out of the house if I didn't go back. But I don't believe her. Anyway, even if she did, I'd just move in with my friend Denise.

THERAPIST: So maybe one goal of therapy is to help you plan what you want to do—in the next few weeks and then in the long run.

JENNA: (*sullenly*) Whatever.

THERAPIST: (*giving her a choice*) Unless you'd rather figure this out on your own.

JENNA: (*indirectly acknowledging that she needs help*) I know Mom is going to make things impossible for me.

THERAPIST: So would another goal be to handle your mom differently?

JENNA: (*sarcastically*) Like that's possible.

THERAPIST: Well, you may be right. Or you may be wrong. Sounds like you're pretty frustrated with her right now.

JENNA: Yeah.

THERAPIST: So maybe you can learn how to talk to her differently. It might have no effect—but then again, it *might* help you get what you want.

JENNA: (*recognizing that the therapist is not going to insist on a goal of going back to work and starting to think more closely about the alternative*) See, I don't really know about work. I definitely don't want to go back to *that* job. But I'm starting to run out of money.

THERAPIST: (*clarifying*) So maybe it would help if we talked about getting a new job, a better job?

JENNA: I guess so.

THERAPIST: (*anticipating that Jenna may feel anxious about the prospect of returning to work*) But, Jenna, if you do decide to go back to work, we'll have to do some preparation. It'd be really important to make it more comfortable for you . . . . Okay?

JENNA: (*Nods.*)

THERAPIST: (*writing down that goal*) Okay, let me see. (*summarizing*) We've got making a decision about work, maybe learning how to talk to your mom differently, maybe learning how to make the next job better . . . Is there any other problem you might want to work on with me?

JENNA: I don't know. Everything sucks.

THERAPIST: For example?

JENNA: (*Sighs.*) All I do all day is lie around. My mom keeps calling me on the phone and nagging me to get up and do stuff. But I have no energy! I call my friends on the phone but I have nothing to say. So I hear all about what this boy did to that girl and how this girl is mad at that girl. Boring!

THERAPIST: Sure sounds like you need more satisfaction in your day.

JENNA: Yeah, but I'm too tired to do anything.

THERAPIST: Oh, then maybe the goal should be "Find satisfying things to do that don't take a lot of energy." Does that sound okay?

JENNA: I guess.

THERAPIST: All right, this looks like a reasonable goal list. Would you be willing to look at it this week and see if there's anything else you want to add—anything else you want to get out of therapy?

JENNA: Okay.

Here the therapist set some initial goals with an unwilling patient. She surprised Jenna by not insisting that Jenna have a goal of immediately returning to work. The therapist believed that Jenna should return to work, but knew they needed to work together to make sure her next work experience was more successful. She knew, however, that if she pushed this goal at this first session, Jenna was likely to refuse to come back to treatment.

In subsequent sessions, the therapist conceptualized difficulties with Jenna that first showed up in goal setting. Her core beliefs were related to helplessness and vulnerability. A key assumption was "If I go back to work, people might humiliate me and I won't be able to handle it." Her strategy, therefore, was to continue to avoid work and, in therapy, to aggressively state that she has no intention of returning to work.

Case Example 8: The Patient Who Doesn't Want to Be in Therapy

Charlie was a 47-year-old manager with obsessive–compulsive personality disorder and no diagnosis on Axis I. A potential difficulty in setting goals became apparent in the first therapy session. Foregoing the usual first-session structure, the therapist suggested that the first topic for discussion could be whether the patient should even engage in treatment. The therapist quickly offered a goal that she believed might be palatable to Charlie to encourage him to remain in therapy.

CHARLIE: I have to tell you, I don't really know why I'm here. It's my wife's idea. She says I need therapy. In fact, she implied she might leave me if I didn't come.

THERAPIST: Then I guess the first thing we should talk about is whether this should be a one-shot deal today or whether you think therapy could help you in some way.

CHARLIE: Well, like I said, it was my wife's idea.

THERAPIST: Can you tell me what she would say if she were here? If I were to say to her, Why do you want Charlie to be in therapy, she'd say . . . ?

CHARLIE: She'd blame her unhappiness on me. She'd say I don't talk to her enough, that I don't "share" things, whatever that means. She'd say I work too hard and I'm no fun anymore.

THERAPIST: Do you think she's right?

CHARLIE: I don't know what she wants from me. She *knows* my job is really demanding. She *likes* the money I make.

THERAPIST: You say she's so unhappy she might leave you?

CHARLIE: Well, she implied that. I don't know for sure.

THERAPIST: And how would you feel about that—if she left?

CHARLIE: I *don't* want her to leave. I really don't. I just want her to get off my back.

THERAPIST: So would your goal in therapy be to figure out what you can do to make things better? Maybe we could figure out some relatively easy things you could do that would be really meaningful to her.

CHARLIE: I don't know. I'll have to think about it.

THERAPIST: Fair enough. (*hypothesizing*) Meanwhile, would there be anything bad about your making some small changes? Would it mean, for example, that she's won and you've lost, or anything like that?

Charlie was feeling somewhat helpless and, as he reported several minutes later, unappreciated and diminished by his wife's criticism of him. Upon questioning, he intimated that he did have a goal of staying married, though initially he did not want to have to make any changes to improve the marriage. His therapist wisely suggested that he think about making some *small* changes but did not ask him to commit to that goal initially. She helped him examine the advantages and disadvantages of that goal so he could draw his own conclusion about whether to modify his behavior toward his wife.

SUMMARY

Patients progress better in therapy when they have a clear picture of what they want and how to get there. Setting specific behavioral objectives is an important part of the process. Many difficulties in treatment may be traced to a lack of mutually agreed-upon goals. In such cases, therapy may not have a clear focus or the therapist and the patient may be implicitly at odds. Often a problem in helping patients set goals is related to the kinds of questions therapists ask or the degree to which they persist when their initial questions are ineffective.

In some instances, however, the problem is related to patients' problematic beliefs and strategies. It is vitally important for therapists to identify such problems, to work with patients to conceptualize these difficulties, and to modify interventions as needed in order to find agreed-upon directions for therapy.

CHAPTER 8

▬▬▬▬

Challenges in Structuring the Session

Cognitive therapists generally implement a standard structure in therapy sessions, one that is designed to deliver treatment as efficiently and effectively as possible. This chapter outlines a recommended structure, then describes how to use and vary standard strategies to adhere to the structure. Dysfunctional assumptions of patients and therapists are presented, along with solutions for common problems therapists encounter in implementing specific structural elements of the session. Finally, conditions under which it is inadvisable to implement a standard structure are described.

STANDARD STRUCTURE

At the beginning of sessions, therapists reestablish rapport and check on changes in patients' symptoms, level of well-being, and functioning. They get the "lay of the land" by asking questions to find out how the week(s) went in general, the high and low points, the problems and successes their patients experienced. They review homework. They determine whether the patient predicts that significant problems might arise before the next session. Collecting this data through both symptom checklists and verbal questioning helps the therapist formulate a strategy for the session. Uppermost in the therapist's mind is:

> ■ "How can I help the patient feel better by the end of this session?"
> ■ "How can I help him/her have a better week(s) (until I see him/her again)?"

This critical first part of the therapy session can be relatively brief if patients are able to concisely provide the information that therapists need—or it may take up to a quarter or even a third of the session, especially if the patient has a great deal of information to impart and/or if the therapist makes an error by failing to interrupt the patient when needed.

In the next part of the session, the therapist prioritizes the agenda with the patient and discusses the first problem. The therapist again collects data about the problem to formulate a strategy. For example, should they do straightforward problem solving? Uncover and examine key dysfunctional cognitions? Focus on relevant skills training? Do something else? Discussion of the problem naturally leads to a homework assignment. This procedure is repeated for the second problem (and the third, if there is time).

Toward the end of the session, the therapist ensures that she and the patient share an understanding of the most important ideas discussed in the session and that they have recorded (on paper or an audiotape) the most important conclusions they have reached and the homework assignment. Finally the therapist elicits feedback.

Therapists sometimes have difficulties instituting or maintaining such a structure for a variety of reasons. As with most therapeutic problems, there may be a practical problem (e.g., the therapist does not interrupt enough), a psychological problem (e.g., the patient has interfering beliefs such as "If I let my therapist structure the session, it will show she's strong and I'm weak") or both. In this chapter, instituting and varying standard strategies to structure the therapy session are presented first. Next, typical maladaptive beliefs of both therapists and patients are discussed. Finally, difficulties with each part of the session structure are presented.

USING AND VARYING STANDARD STRATEGIES TO STRUCTURE SESSIONS

Many problems in structuring sessions arise because of therapist error. The therapist may fail to socialize the patient adequately, to negotiate the structure when indicated, to pace the session effectively, or to interrupt the patient when needed. It is important to educate patients so that they will understand that structuring sessions enables therapists to help them solve their problems most efficiently and effectively.

Patients who were previously in relatively unstructured treatment may initially find the structured approach of cognitive therapy unsettling. But if they do not have interfering assumptions, they are often willing to experiment with a different approach, especially if their therapists are careful to say that they will ask for feedback and collaboratively determine the usefulness of structure to the patient. Using the "Preparing for Therapy" worksheet (J. Beck, 2005) is helpful to many patients because it enables them to gather their thoughts and recognize what will be important for them to express to their therapist at the beginning of the session.

Negotiating the Structure of Sessions

Sometimes therapists need to negotiate the structure of the session with patients. Some patients have virtually no one else in their lives to whom they can speak about their problems. Other patients cannot concentrate on evaluating their cognitions or solving problems until they unburden themselves to the therapist. Patients such as these often benefit from a period of time at the beginning of sessions to speak without interruption. Having conceptualized this need, therapists can make a collaborative agreement with patients to allow them to speak for the first 10 or 15 minutes of every session (at least initially). At the end of this time, therapists should step in to summarize the most important points the patient has made, check to make sure that they have an accurate understanding of the patient's report, and then use the patient's soliloquy to create important agenda items. They can then institute a more standard structure for the rest of the session: doing a mood check, bridging the session, discussing agenda items, and so on. It is important, however, for therapists to establish that such a variation is necessary and not to assume that a patient will not benefit from the standard structure from the beginning.

Pacing

Another essential skill for effective structuring of sessions is pacing. Therapists need to continuously monitor the time remaining in a session and tactfully guide discussion so that they can help patients feel better by the end of the session and prepare them to have a better week. It is useful to have two clocks in the therapy office so that both therapists and patients can take responsibility for monitoring how the time is spent. Therapists should wrap up the discussion of the last problem 5 to 10 minutes before the end of the session. Doing so enables patients and therapists to arrive at closure on a problem (or to collaboratively agree to continue discussing the problem at the next session), to review and record both the most important conclusions from the session and the homework assignment, and to discuss patients' feedback about the session.

Interrupting

Therapists cannot pace sessions and accomplish therapeutic goals unless they tactfully interrupt patients. Patients initially do not know what the therapist needs to know to help them effectively. Some patients (and therapists) think the therapist needs to know every detail about the patient's history and about each problem to be helpful. Or that they need to know everything that has been challenging to a patient or has been on his or her mind. In fact, therapists generally need to have enough information to conceptualize which problem is the most important one to work on, and then in the context of solving the problem, what background information is most important, and which cognitions and behaviors are most essential to modify.

Therefore it is important for therapists to gently interrupt patients—for example, by saying: "Can I interrupt you for a moment? I want to make sure I understand what you're saying"; or "Can I just ask you a question about this?"; or "Sorry to break in, but I need to know . . . ." Patients who are distressed by interruptions will usually display a change in affect, body language, or tone of voice. Chapters 4 and 5 describe what to do in such cases. If therapists are unsure of the effect of their interruptions on the patient, they can simply ask:

> ■ "I'm sorry to keep interrupting you, but it's important for me [to get a full picture/to get a sense of the range of your problems/to find out what was most distressing to you]. Does it bother you too much?"

If the patient replies in the affirmative, the therapist can negotiate the structure with the patient or see whether the patient is willing to tolerate the interruptions—and then determine at the end of the session if a change is needed for the following session.

DYSFUNCTIONAL ASSUMPTIONS OF PATIENTS AND THERAPISTS

Typical assumptions of patients that interfere with implementing a standard structure often reflect dysfunctional ideas patients have about themselves, about their therapist, and about being in therapy:

> • "If my therapist interrupts me it means she doesn't care/doesn't want to hear what's on my mind/is trying to control me/is demeaning me."
> • "If my therapist interrupts me, she'll miss out on crucial information that she needs to help me/won't understand me."
> • "If my therapist structures the session, I'll feel uncomfortable/have to reveal myself/have to face and work on my problems."

Therapists, too, sometimes make maladaptive assumptions:

- "If I interrupt the patient, I'll miss out on important information."
- "If I structure the session, I'll damage our alliance."

Therapists with these kinds of assumptions need to evaluate their ideas and do experiments to test them. If therapists do miss important information, they can engage in more thorough questioning. If the alliance is damaged, they can work to repair it.

When patients are distressed, they tend to focus on either the most recent upsetting event or on the event that distressed them most during the week. Sometimes these topics *are* of primary importance. However, unless therapists interrupt patients, they often do not have sufficient data to make this determination. *Failure to interrupt patients deprives them of the opportunity to think through what will help them the most so they can get the greatest benefit from the session.*

Harriet, for example, came to session very upset; she had just had another fight with her adult daughter. Had her therapist not interrupted Harriet, he may not have found out until the end of the session, if at all, that she was facing a far more pressing problem: her public assistance benefits were about to be terminated because Harriet had been avoiding filling out the necessary forms and meeting with her caseworker.

Sometimes therapists benefit from rehearsing adaptive responses to their dysfunctional assumptions—for example,

"Interrupting this patient feels uncomfortable to me. But I know from prior experience that *not* interrupting him means we don't get very much accomplished. I can try interrupting and see what happens. If he becomes distressed, I can always apologize and tell him that I'm interrupting because it's very important to me that I really help him solve his problems. On the other hand, it might not be a problem at all."

SOLVING PROBLEMS IN STRUCTURING THE THERAPY SESSION

Problems in implementing standard structure are presented in this chapter and in Chapter 9. This section discusses difficulties that arise at the beginning of sessions (while doing mood checks with patients, setting the agenda, bridging the therapy session, and prioritizing agenda items) and at the end of sessions (while summarizing and eliciting feedback). The next chapter describes problems from the middle part of a standard session: discussing agenda topics and setting homework.

It is important to note that the standard elements at the beginning of a therapy session are presented here as separate items. In reality, experienced therapists often blend these elements together.

Mood Check

It is valuable to have patients fill out standard symptom checklists, such as the Beck Depression Inventory (Beck et al., 1961), the Anxiety Inventory (Beck, Epstein, Brown & Steer, 1988), and the Hopelessness Scale (Beck, Weissman, Lester & Trexler, 1974), before each session. Or patients can rate their mood on a scale of 0–10 or 0–100, or simply rate their distress as low, medium, or high. In addition, therapists should elicit a subjective report about how the patient felt in the past week compared to other weeks. Sometimes, though, patients become distressed at having to rate their mood. The following example illustrates how the therapist had to forego a standard mood check to keep a tenuous therapeutic alliance intact.

Although Andrea grudgingly filled out symptom checklists and other forms at the initial evaluation, she flatly refused to complete them again before the first therapy session ("I absolutely won't fill them out"). Deciding that this problem was of minor importance compared to Andrea's other problems, her therapist withdrew the request and tried to get the information in other ways.

THERAPIST: Did you fill out the [depression and anxiety] forms?

ANDREA: (*flatly*) No.

THERAPIST: I'd like to get an idea of how you've been feeling since the evaluation. Could you fill them out after the session?

ANDREA: I *really* don't want to. They really don't apply to me.

THERAPIST: Then let's figure out another way for you to rate your mood. Can you tell me, if 100 is the most depressed you've ever felt and 0 means you don't feel depressed at all, where would you rate your mood in general this week?

ANDREA: (*irritably*) I don't know. (*pause*) I hate having to do that. It seems so artificial.

THERAPIST: Would you rather tell me in your own words how you're feeling this week compared to other weeks?

ANDREA: I don't know. I feel lousy, that's how I feel.

THERAPIST: (*empathically*) I'm sorry—sounds like you had another bad week.

ANDREA: Yeah.

THERAPIST: (*trying to get more specific information*) What was the worst part of the week?

ANDREA: It was all bad.

THERAPIST: Can you give me an example of *one* bad time? (*providing a choice*) Would it have been in the last couple of days? Or toward the beginning of the week?

ANDREA: (*Thinks.*) I told you, everything was bad.

THERAPIST: (*trying the opposite tact*) Where there any times this week that weren't as bad as other times? (*providing a choice*). Did you watch anything good on television? Have a good meal?

ANDREA: I watched [a reality show]. That was pretty good.

THERAPIST: So there was at least one slightly brighter hour in your week. (*conversationally*) Are you going to watch it again this week?

ANDREA: Yeah, I always do.

THERAPIST: That's good. (*providing the rationale for a mood check*) You know, one reason I ask your how your mood was during the week is to find out what was good—so you can do more of it. And what was bad—so we can try to fix it. In general, do you think your mood this week was as bad as it was, say, last month? Or are there better points now? Are you able to enjoy shows like [the reality show] more?

ANDREA: (*thinks*) I don't think so. I don't see much difference. Maybe a little worse now.

THERAPIST: Okay, well I'd like to continue to keep tabs on your mood at the beginning of every session, so I'll know if we seem to be going in the right direction or if we need to change something about the therapy. Okay?

ANDREA: (*reluctantly*) Okay.

Here the therapist was flexible and compromising. Had she pushed Andrea to rate her mood, their tenuous therapeutic alliance probably would have deteriorated. At the beginning of the second therapy session, the therapist again gently evaluates the patient's willingness to rate her mood.

THERAPIST: What do you think, if I ask you to rate your mood, will it irritate you?

ANDREA: Yeah, probably.

THERAPIST: Then I won't ask you today, but can you tell me what it *means* to you that I'm asking about your mood?

ANDREA: It's frustrating. I can't just give you a short answer about how I feel. It's very complicated.

THERAPIST: Do you think it's important for me to understand, even if it is complicated?

ANDREA: No. No. I'd rather talk about something else.

THERAPIST: That's okay. (*changing the subject to preserve the alliance*) Can we set the agenda? What problem do you want my help in solving today?

Refusing to rate her mood was just one difficulty Andrea presented. She also changed the subject when her therapist asked her to describe a typical day in the past week. She insisted on setting an agenda that included only a description of the many traumas she had experienced growing up in her "dysfunctional" family. Andrea's difficulties in focusing on her current mood, functioning, and problems stemmed from her assumption, "If I talk about my [current] problems, I'll feel terrible." Her therapist initially skipped a standard mood check. Over time, as Andrea experienced *relief* from discussing her current problems in therapy, she became more cooperative in session in general, including allowing her therapist to do a standard mood check.

Setting an Initial Agenda

Therapists may ask patients for problems for the agenda toward the very beginning of sessions, then gather additional topics as they arise during the bridge. Following the bridge, the therapist may summarize the agenda items gleaned thus far and ascertain whether patients have other items they would like to discuss.

Asking many patients what they would like to put on the agenda results in problem-oriented topics. But asking some patients a general question, such as "What do you want to talk about this week?" or "What do you think we should discuss?", sometimes leads to agenda items that do not help the patient progress. With these patients it is better to ask:

> ■ "What problems do you want my help in solving today?"

This question, however, is still too open-ended for some patients, particularly those who are lower functioning. The therapist may need to take the lead in setting the agenda. (e.g., "Asher, is it okay if we check on how you're managing at home and taking your medicine and getting along with others? Let me know if there's anything else for our agenda.")

A number of difficulties can arise when trying to set an initial agenda with patients with challenging problems. They may:

- Fail to respond.
- Reveal a reluctance to be in therapy.
- Avoid naming an important problem.
- Describe a problem instead of naming it.
- Become overwhelmed as they name too many problems.

These difficulties are discussed below.

When Patients Say, "I Don't Know"

Sometimes an "I don't know" response is genuine; patients may feel so overwhelmed by a myriad of difficulties or by intense emotion that they need the therapist to ask more questions to help them specify what they need to work on. Sometimes a failure to respond indicates a problem in the alliance: (e.g., "If I make myself vulnerable by telling my therapist my problems, she'll hurt me"). Sometimes it reflects the patient's strategy of avoidance: (e.g., "If I put 'getting a job' on the agenda, I'll have to start trying to find one—which I don't want to do").

Case Example

Arthur, a chronically depressed 31-year-old man who is unemployed and still living with his parents, initially only wanted to discuss existential issues. He is initially unengaged and obviously reluctant to set an agenda. His therapist shifts into a review of his week to try to engage him and identify important problems for the agenda.

THERAPIST: What problem do you want help with today?

ARTHUR: (*Hesitates.*) I don't know.

THERAPIST: (*looking back at the notes from the previous session*) Do you think we should talk about the problem with your parents? Or with not getting much satisfaction from your life?

ARTHUR: I guess.

THERAPIST: Anything else?

ARTHUR: Not really.

THERAPIST: (*Moves to bridge from last session.*) Okay, let's get caught up. What happened this week I should know about? How was your week?

After discussing items on the bridge, the therapist makes a second attempt at establishing an agenda.

THERAPIST: (*summarizing*) Okay, sounds as if things are still pretty bad with your parents but there were times this week that you felt a little bit less depressed. Which one do you think we should talk more about now? Or is there another problem that you want to work on?

When Patients Are Reluctant to Set an Agenda Because They Do Not Want to Engage in Therapy

Arthur, the patient discussed above, is still reluctant to set an agenda because he does not want to be in treatment. His therapist has to present a strong case for why, from the patient's point of view, he might want to engage in therapy.

ARTHUR: You know, I don't really want to talk about anything. I don't want to be here at all.

THERAPIST: So it was hard for you to come in today?

ARTHUR: Yeah, but I had to. My parents insisted.

THERAPIST: So you had no choice. You know, if I were you, I'd be feeling pretty resentful.

ARTHUR: Yeah, I mean, therapy was *their* idea, not mine.

THERAPIST: Do you feel like they try to push you around a lot? Or is it just therapy that they've insisted on?

ARTHUR: No, they do it a lot.

THERAPIST: Can you give me some more examples?

Here the therapist engages the patient by empathizing with his reluctance and, instead of setting an initial agenda, allows him to vent. Next, the therapist engages the patient by phrasing an agenda item in a way that is palatable to him:

THERAPIST: Sounds as if your parents are really trying to control you—not only telling you what you need to do and what you can't do—but also making you feel so bad. Do you want to talk about what you can do so they can't control your mood so much?

ARTHUR: (*appearing more engaged*) What do you mean?

THERAPIST: Seems to me that you're going around feeling pretty angry a lot of the time, especially when you're thinking about how much they pressure you and criticize you. (*pause*) Would you like to know how to be in control of your own mood? Not be so angry—unless it suits *you*?

ARTHUR: I'm still not sure what you mean.

THERAPIST: Well, why don't we put "being in control of my own mood" and "problem with parents" on the agenda to talk about today. (*pause*) Before we get to those, is there anything else you want to work on?

When Patients Avoid Putting an Important Problem on the Agenda

Sometimes patients, especially those who tend to be avoidant, put items on the agenda but do not bring up the most crucial problem.

Case Example

Rosa had chronic, long-standing problems with her brother. Because he lived out of state and because she generally avoided contact with him, problems with him arose infrequently. Although Rosa wanted to talk about him, her therapist conceptualized that it was more important to focus on helping Rosa find a job, since her limited funds would soon be exhausted.

THERAPIST: So what problems do you want to work on today?

ROSA: This fight I had with my brother, I guess. He was bugging me to visit my parents so I told him off.

THERAPIST: Anything else?

ROSA: (*Thinks.*) Uh, if we have time, my apartment is such a mess.

THERAPIST: (*mentioning an ongoing problem*) And how about your progress in looking for a job?

ROSA: Yeah, I guess.

Difficulty with this patient may arise when it is time to *prioritize* the problems on the agenda.

THERAPIST: Okay, let's figure out how to spend our time. There's the problem with your brother and your apartment and finding a job. Which do you think we should start with?

ROSA: My brother. He really upset me.

THERAPIST: I wonder, Rosa, if we should talk about a job first. It concerns me that your unemployment insurance is going to run out this month. Do you have a back-up plan in case you don't have a job yet?

Here the therapist directs the discussion toward a problem that she deems more pressing. Instead of collaboratively making the decision to talk about the job, she just starts talking about it—seeking information. If the patient objects, the therapist might ask for her automatic thoughts about discussing the problem.

When Patients Start Describing a Problem Instead of Just Naming It

Therapists need to socialize patients to therapy, in essence, to teach them how to get maximal benefit from treatment. Part of the socialization process is teaching them to name, not to describe their problems when setting the agenda. Therapists often have to interrupt and model this skill for the patient.

Case Example

Anita, a 36-year-old homemaker, started talking even before she sat down: "It was such a terrible week. My husband, you know he got laid off last month, he is so irritable all the time. He's constantly complaining, too. Like last night, I got home a little late from having coffee with my friends and he was really upset. He is so set in his ways. He wants dinner on the table by 6:00 and if it isn't he . . . ."

Had the therapist let the patient continue, she would not have found out other problems that were more important. Sometimes therapists must interrupt several times:

THERAPIST: Anita, let me interrupt for a minute. So we want to put the problem with your husband. . . .

ANITA: . . . gets bent out of shape. If dinner is late, it just seems to throw him for a loop, . . .

THERAPIST: (*holding up a finger*) Anita, sorry to interrupt you . . .

ANITA: Then he gets all sarcastic . . .

THERAPIST: (*gently waving her hand*) Anita! Wait a minute. This is really important. Can we call this "Problem with Bob?" Can you write that down on this piece of paper? I want to hear about that in a few minutes, but first I need to know how you're feeling and how your week was and what other problems you might be having. Now, can you tell me in just a couple of sentences what your mood was like in general this week?

Here the therapist had to be persistent or she would not have been able to get the information she needed to plan treatment for that session. Asking the patient to write down the agenda item is not a common practice, but the therapist had to be creative in getting Anita to refocus her attention. It helped interrupt Anita's flow of speech and allowed her to switch gears so she could reflect on the therapist's questions. Had Anita then had a negative reaction to the therapist's behavior, the therapist could have followed the suggestions in Chapters 4 and 5, on the therapeutic relationship. And as mentioned previously, failure to interrupt Anita may have deprived her of the opportunity to think through what was most important to her to talk about in session. She might not, therefore, have felt better by the end of the session nor had a better week.

When Patients Put Too Many Problems on the Agenda

Sometimes patients start blurting out problems as soon as they enter their therapists' office, overwhelming themselves and their therapist. The therapist needs to interrupt and summarize, grouping related problems under one topic name.

Case Example

PATIENT: I had such a hard week. I don't even know where to start. I'm having that problem with my neighbor. Again. Again! He's making my life miserable. And then there's this thing at work. Wanda—I told you about her before—she's been getting worse, always telling me what to do even though she's not my supervisor. She's got seniority but what I do is my business not hers. And Simon [boyfriend], I don't know what's up with him. He runs so hot and cold. He said something this week that was so hurtful, but then he apologized right away, I don't know. And I think I'm running out of money. I don't even know how much I have in the bank, and I'm maxed out on my credit cards and I got a letter from a collection agency this week. And my mother is driving me crazy, calling me all the time, like she expects me to always be at her beck and call. And I'm feeling lousy, I think I'm coming down with a cold but I can't afford to miss any more work or I think they might fire me. And my roommate, I think she's stealing money from me. And she won't clean up her share. The kitchen is always messy. It's disgusting.

THERAPIST: (*interrupting and summarizing*) So, let's see what we should work on first. There's a problem with money, there are problems with relationships, and a problem if you get sick. If we only had time to work on one problem, which one do you think would make the biggest difference?

PATIENT: I don't know. I'm so mad at my neighbor. And my roommate. (*thinks*) My roommate, I guess. I can just ignore my neighbor, pretend I don't see him.

THERAPIST: Okay, we can start with your roommate. If we have time for another problem, what would it be?

Making a Bridge between Sessions

In this portion of the session, therapists gather additional information they need to set and prioritize a full agenda and plan the session effectively. They may need to do some or all of the following, though not necessarily in any prescribed order:

- Assess patients' current functioning through a brief review of their week (including the best and worst parts of the week).
- Determine whether there are critical upcoming events.
- Discuss negative reactions to the previous session (when relevant).
- Check on adherence to medication (when relevant).
- Review homework (including, when relevant, cravings for and/or use of alcohol/drugs, and frequency of impulsive behaviors, etc.).
- Assess patients' level of commitment to reach goals (when relevant).
- Assess patients' degree of belief in core beliefs (when relevant).

These topics are described below.

Review of the Week

Patients vary in the degree to which they spontaneously relate important data about their week (or about the period since they last had contact with the therapist). Some, even those without challenging problems, report far too little; others report far too much. In order to conceptualize how best to help the patient at a given session, therapists need to get a broad overview of how the week went and also to probe for specific information about when the patient was most distressed. Therapists may recognize important problems to put on the agenda from the patient's report. It is important to note that some patients may not spontaneously report problems in essential areas. It may be helpful to quickly review specific aspects of their functioning to see whether a problem has arisen that should be put on the agenda.

Case Example

Laura, a long-term patient with rapid-cycling bipolar disorder, came to therapy once a week when she was in crisis, less often when she was doing better, and once every 6 weeks to 2 months when she was relatively stable. Her therapist recognized Laura's pattern of putting on the agenda only the problem that was most distressing to her on the day of her appointment. Occasionally there were other crucial problems that Laura failed to mention. Therefore, at the beginning of each session, her therapist quickly went down a checklist with Laura of the critical areas in her life: "How are things going with your boyfriend? With your daughter? How many times did you miss taking your medicine since I saw you last? When did you see your psychiatrist? What did she say? Are you able to keep up with the housework? How are things with your mother and sister? Are you still reading the Bible most days? Are you eating regularly? Sleeping? Getting outside for a walk? Doing errands?" Failure to discover and work on problems promptly often contributed to Laura's decline.

Therapists should also inquire about the *positive* aspects of their patients' week. Doing so allows the therapist to reinforce patients for engaging in functional behavior and changing their thinking—and to reinforce the idea that patients impacted their mood by thinking and behaving in a different way. Reviewing positive events can also help patients see that their lives are not unremittingly negative. Finally, therapists can collect positive data to use later in that session or in future sessions to counter the patient's dysfunctional core beliefs (see Chapter 13).

Anticipating positive responses, Laura's therapist, for example, also asked her questions such as "How was church last Sunday? How is your dog doing? Are you enjoying the mild weather? Are you making headway on the scarf you're knitting for your daughter? What did you do this week that was enjoyable?"

Anticipating Future Difficulties

To set an effective agenda it is important to ascertain whether significant problems may arise before the next therapy session. Therapists might ask:

> ■ "Is there anything coming up before I see you again that I should know?"

If patients bring up potential problems, therapists can assess with them whether discussion of these problems should take precedence over problems that arose in the past week. For example, Jerry and his therapist decided that discussing how he could handle an upcoming visit from a family member should take precedence over a distressing incident the day before with a bill collector. Making sure that potential upcoming problems are on the agenda should also avert, at least some of the time, patients bringing up important problems toward the end of the session—for example, "But I forgot to tell you that my landlord is threatening to evict me in a few days!"

Negative Reactions to the Previous Session

When patients have expressed a negative reaction at the end of the previous session, it may be important to discuss this problem at the very beginning of the next therapy session, as described in Chapters 4 and 5, even before doing a mood check or setting the agenda. On the other hand, therapists may judge, unless they have promised the patient otherwise, that it is better to delay this discussion until later in the session when they predict the patient may feel more engaged and the alliance is more firmly reestablished.

Adherence to Medication

Until patients display a consistent pattern of medication adherence, it is beneficial to check, at the beginning of the session, how consistently they are taking their psychotropic medication. "Did you take your medicine this week?" invariably leads to a "yes" answer. More specific questions often yield important information:

> ■ "How many days this week were you able to take your medicine exactly as prescribed?"

A variation of this question is:

■ "How many days did you skip taking some of your medicine?"

If the patient was not fully compliant, the therapist can put this problem on the agenda.

Review of Homework

Sometimes review of homework is brief: patients report it was helpful, are able to concisely describe what they learned or how they benefited from doing it, and quickly decide with the therapist whether to continue the assignments. At the other end of the spectrum are the situations in which a review of the homework should occupy most of the therapy session because the homework addresses the central problems and beliefs for which the patient continues to need help. In this case, "review of homework" should probably become a topic for the agenda, so the therapist can continue the bridge between sessions and help the patient prioritize the agenda. There is often a fine balance between reviewing homework assignments fully enough and still retaining enough time to discuss agenda items unrelated to the homework.

Marjorie's homework had been to test her belief, "If I express my opinion to people [husband, sister, friend, neighbor], they'll get mad at me and hurt me in some way." During the bridge, the therapist ascertained that Marjorie had done several behavioral experiments, some of which had gone well, some of which had not. The patient agreed to wait until they had prioritized a full agenda to discuss the homework more fully. Indeed Marjorie and her therapist decided that a problem with Marjorie's work was even more pressing, and so they subsequently devoted some time to reviewing the behavioral experiments but agreed to discuss them more fully at the next session.

When reviewing homework, the therapist needs to find out the extent to which the patient fulfilled the assignments. As with the medication issue, the question "Did you read your therapy notes?" often yields less valuable information than:

■ "How often did you (or were you able to) read them?"

Benjamin's therapist asked him how often he had driven to the supermarket during the past week, an important exercise on his agoraphobia hierarchy. At first Benjamin reported that he had gone "most of the time." Upon further questioning, he revealed that he had only gone twice, which had not been enough for him to practice his adaptive coping techniques and gain mastery of the task. This was important information for the therapist to know as she planned the session.

Research shows that patients who do homework have better outcomes than those who do not (Persons, Burns, & Perloff, 1988). Therefore therapists should stress the importance of doing homework and to review with patients who did not complete their assignments what got in the way (see Chapter 9).

The beginning of the session is also a good time to check on substance use, when relevant.

> ■ "How many days this week did you [have a drink]? What was the most you [drank] in a day? The least? The average?"

When working with a patient who abuses substances, it is also important to ask about the frequency and severity of *urges*. Even if patients did not drink or use drugs, discussion of how they handled their urges can indicate whether this topic should also go on the agenda. Also, patients who are reluctant to provide honest data about the extent of their substance use may be willing to own up to having urges, leading to an important discussion.

Commitment to Reach a Goal

If patients do not do their homework, seem ambivalent about reaching their goals, or do not focus on solving problems, the beginning of the therapy session is a good place to assess how strongly they still want to reach their goals. The therapist might say: "Tell me, your goal to manage better at home, how much do you really want to do that right now?" If the patient's commitment is low, the therapist can either focus on other agenda items or see if the patient is willing to set for an agenda item a discussion of the advantages and disadvantages of working toward this goal at this point.

Selena, for example, was a 22-year-old woman with anorexia and depression who was living at home with her parents, attending school part time and working part time. Although she was recovering from her eating disorder, at times she still displayed significant restriction and overexercise. She tended to minimize and offer rationalizations to justify her dysfunctional behavior. Her therapist helped Selena to be more forthcoming and to engage in less self-defeating justification of her dysfunctional behavior by asking her how much she still wanted to achieve her goal of independence at the beginning of each session.

Strength of Core Belief

Once the therapist and the patient start modifying a core belief, the beginning of the therapy session is a good place to monitor the degree to which the patient still believes it at both the intellectual and the emotional level (see Chapter 13).

> ■ "So we've been working on this idea that you're 'nothing.' How much do you believe that right now? At an intellectual level? At a gut level? When did you believe it most this week? When did you believe it least?"

This brief discussion can provide important data to be used later in the session as therapist and patient discuss evidence contrary to the patient's core belief and supportive of the new, more adaptive belief. Such a discussion also reminds patients and therapists to be alert for the activation of the belief during the session and for determining whether the belief underlies the problems on the agenda.

Prioritizing the Agenda

Some patients have a clear idea of which agenda items are most important to discuss. Some patients, though, have difficulty figuring out what will help them the most—or actively avoid choosing to discuss their most critical problems. As mentioned previously, the therapist reflects on two time frames: What is most likely to help the patient feel better by the end of the session? What is most likely to help the patient most during the coming week(s)?

When patients are overwhelmed by a number of problems, the therapist can try a variety of techniques. Some patients are able to select an important problem without much guidance:

> ■ "It sounds like there are a lot of things distressing you. That must be hard . . . . Given that we'll probably only have time to work on one or two of them, can you tell me which is most important to you?"

For other patients, it is useful to summarize the problems in groups:

> ■ "So there are problems [at work, problems with your husband and children, and problems with feeling anxious and lonely]. Where do you want to start?"

Or the therapist can be more directive, though still in a collaborative way, if he or she has a clear sense of what is most important:

> ■ "You know, some of these things are pretty chronic problems. I wonder whether we ought to discuss [your mother's visit] this week first. It seems like in the past that has been pretty bad for you. (pause) What do you think?"

Discussing Problems on the Agenda and Setting Homework

These elements are the heart of the therapy session and are discussed in detail in the next chapter.

Summarizing

During the therapy session, it is essential to get a sense of the patients' emotional experience in the moment and of their understanding of the session content. Therapists need to know what patients are thinking and how they are reacting—which is often difficult to gauge unless the therapist directly asks questions such as:

> ■ "Can you summarize what we just talked about?"
> ■ "What's the main message here?"
> ■ "What do you think my point is?"

It may then be important to ask questions such as:

> ■ "What do you think about that? ... How much do you believe that?"
> ■ "How do you feel about what we've just been discussing?"

If patients summarize accurately but seem doubtful, therapists should invite patients' skepticism and elicit their automatic thoughts:

THERAPIST: Can you summarize? What do you think I'm saying here?

PATIENT: That the way to feel better is to get more active.

THERAPIST: Exactly! And what do you think about that?

PATIENT: I don't know. I've tried to do things like you're suggesting before, but nothing really helps.

THERAPIST: So your thought is "If I get more active, it won't help." And are you feeling hopeless?

PATIENT: Yeah.

THERAPIST: How much do you believe this idea right now: "If I get more active, it won't help"?

Therapists can then use standard Socratic questioning and set up behavioral experiments so patients can test their assumptions. If therapists fail to probe for patients' reactions, they may not uncover their skepticism— and therefore will not have an opportunity to address it.

If the patient's summary is not accurate or adaptive, therapists can offer a mild correction—and, if patients have become upset, they can decrease their distress.

THERAPIST: Can you summarize what we've just talked about?

PATIENT: (*irritated*) Well, *you're* saying that I *just* have to have a thicker skin so my dysfunctional family won't make me fall apart.

THERAPIST: Well, that's partly right, but I absolutely *don't* think it's a matter of just developing a thicker skin. (*pause*) I think *we* have to work *together* to help you stand up to them—if you want. And to learn how to ignore them more—so they won't be able to upset you as much. (*pause*) What do you think about that?

Therapy Notes

Having devised a good summary, therapists often ask patients to write it down, or offer to write it down for them. Patients forget much of what they hear in a doctor's office (for a description of their difficulties, see Meichenbaum & Turk, 1987). Therefore therapists ought to assume that the same is true for their psychotherapy patients. To help therapists become aware of what is important for patients to recall, they can continually ask themselves throughout the therapy session:

■ "What do I wish [this patient] would remember this week?"

The therapist then helps the patient to create idiosyncratically devised therapy notes. These notes may contain adaptive ideas (responses to dysfunctional cognitions or conclusions the patient has drawn), instructions to change their behavior, or homework assignments. Patients or therapists can write these important reminders on index cards, in a notebook, or on paper. Therapists can then photocopy these notes. (To avoid photocopying, therapists can obtain no-carbon-required paper from a printer, either full size, or designed to resemble a prescription pad.) Alternatively, therapists and patients can record these "therapy notes" on an audiotape.

Patients will then have the opportunity to review the most important conclusions they drew during the session at home (both in the coming weeks and even after they finish their course of treatment). They benefit from reading their therapy notes on a regular basis (e.g., at breakfast and dinner) and also on a PRN (as-needed) basis. Therapists sometimes need to be creative in helping patients who cannot read and do not have access to a cassette player. Patients can draw pictures or symbols to help them remember or they can ask carefully selected people to read their notes to them.

These therapy notes are really the patient's "take-home therapy." It is vitally important to motivate patients to read their notes regularly to facilitate changing their cognitions and behavior. (For more on this topic, see J. Beck, 2001.)

Feedback

As described in Chapters 4 and 5, it is important to elicit feedback *during* a session if patients' automatic thoughts about their therapist, about therapy, or about themselves are interfering with collaboratively working together to solve the patients' problems. Some patients, however, mask their displeasure during the session, which is why it is important to ask for feedback at the end of the session:

> ■ "What did you think about today's session?"
> ■ "Was there anything that bothered you about this session?"
> ■ "Anything you thought I got wrong?"
> ■ "Anything you'd like to change at our next session?"

Chapters 4 and 5 described how to deal with patients who do not reveal their discomfort and with patients who reveal their discomfort vociferously. It is important to leave sufficient time to discuss negative feedback at the end of a session. If therapists run out of time, they need to apologize for not being able to discuss the problem at the moment and motivate patients to return for their next appointment, even if they are still distressed:

> ■ "I'm really glad you told me that [you feel as if I'm taking your family's side in this—I never meant to imply that]. This is *really* important and I'm sorry we don't have time to talk about it now. Would you be willing to talk about this *first* thing next session?"

WHEN IT IS IMPORTANT *NOT* TO STRUCTURE THE SESSION

Sometimes the negative assumptions therapists make about structuring the session are indeed accurate. Interrupting a patient may lead the therapist to miss out on important information. The therapist may want to pursue a topic at the beginning of a session while the patient's core beliefs are activated instead of initially setting a full agenda. Patients may need to unburden themselves before they are emotionally ready to problem-solve. And adhering to a strict structure may damage the therapeutic alliance. When therapists believe, based on data they observe, that these consequences are likely, they should reduce the level of structure, at least initially.

Some patients may simply be unwilling to let the therapist direct the session, even when a lack of direction seems to the therapist to be detrimental. Often therapists have no choice but to compromise. Less drastically, they can negotiate for an unstructured period of time within the session, followed by a more structured period of time within that session. More drastically, they may need to offer a number of unstructured sessions: "Dora, you know you may be right. Maybe you *would* be better off with less structured sessions. What do you think of this? Let's make the next three sessions unstructured. If you're feeling significantly better at the end of that time, we'll know we should continue on that way. If you're *not* feeling significantly better, we'll know that something needs to change. Maybe then we can experiment with focusing on solving problems. (*pause*) What do you think?"

SUMMARY

Following a standard structure is sometimes difficult and the therapist must be careful to vary therapy so that it is acceptable to the patient. Providing rationales for structure, testing how much interrupting patients can tolerate, and modifying patients' (and therapists') assumptions often enables therapists to structure sessions in a way that leads to optimally efficient and effective treatment. Structure usually helps maximize the short time allotted for treatment and facilitates pursuit of ongoing goals, gradual learning of psychological and behavioral skills, and retention of important information in long-term memory. A slavish devotion to following a set structure can be maladaptive and it is not necessarily beneficial to every patient to follow a set pattern of activities at every session. Structure is a means to an end and the standard structure should be assessed for its own "goodness of fit" for the patients.

CHAPTER 9

Challenges in Solving Problems and in Homework

A central tenet of cognitive therapy is that it is not sufficient for patients to talk about their difficulties in therapy sessions. They need to focus on ways of solving their problems *in* session and then try to implement solutions *between* sessions. The therapist's first challenge is to get patients to focus on an important problem and describe it to the therapist, along with their associated dysfunctional cognitions. The second challenge is to get patients to adopt a problem-solving frame of mind so that they can actively collaborate with their therapist to respond to interfering cognitions, when applicable, and devise a solution to the problem. Patients, especially those with challenging problems, vary in their ability and willingness to do so, at least initially.

Some difficulties in solving problems were addressed in the previous chapter: patients who are reluctant to set an agenda and name problems, bring up too many problems, or avoid bringing up important problems. Other difficulties related to the therapeutic relationship were addressed in Chapters 4 and 5: patients who, when their therapist tries to focus on problem solving, claim that their therapist does not understand them, or that the therapy is not right for them, or who become angry at the therapist.

Additional problems are addressed in this chapter. First, case examples illustrate how patients differ in their approach to solving their difficulties and doing homework. The following sections describe how to use and vary standard strategies to help patients solve problems and follow through with homework assignments. Next patients' typical dysfunctional beliefs are described and interventions are suggested. An extended case example then illustrates many of the strategies presented in this chapter. Finally, guidelines for what therapists should do when patients are not progressing and for when problem solving is inappropriate are offered.

Patients' Responses to Working on a Problem

The following examples illustrate how four patients differ in their approach to a problem. They share a common goal: to clean and organize their homes. However, they also share the same problem: they spend much of the day sitting on the couch watching television. In the second therapy session, each expresses a different view about solving this problem.

- The "easy" patient clearly describes the problem and engages in problem solving. During the session he thinks, "It's good we're working on this. [My therapist] seems to understand that I'm feeling overwhelmed. I probably can do some of these small things this week. I can see how it'll help." Although he has a belief that he can't cope, he is willing to suspend judgment and try the assignment.
- Challenging patient 1 outwardly agrees to try some small tasks as a behavioral experiment but is thinking, "I know I'm going to feel too tired and too down to do this. Even if I try, I won't be able to do it very well." Underneath, he has a strong belief that he is helpless and incapable.
- Challenging patient 2 continually changes the subject when his therapist tries to engage him in problem solving. He is thinking, "I don't want to do these things." Underneath is his belief, "If I have to do things I don't want to do, it diminishes me."
- Challenging patient 3 states that he is unwilling to even describe the problem, saying it is trivial and unimportant compared to the major problems in his life. He is thinking, "[My therapist] will try to make me do things." Underneath are his beliefs that others will try to control him and he is weak if he listens to them.

Even if the therapist is able to get patients to focus on a problem, do problem-solving, agree to a homework assignment, and actually *do* the assignment, the difficulty may not be resolved. Each patient above had a different perspective on the experience that influenced his motivation and willingness to engage in *further* problem solving and behavioral change.

- Easy patient: "That was really good! I was able to do all these things. I guess I did have enough energy. Therapy is really helping."
- Challenging patient 1: "I did these things but I didn't do them very well and now I'm exhausted. Therapy isn't helping. I'll never feel better."
- Challenging patient 2: "I did all these things but I hated doing them. It's not fair that I should have to spend my life in drudgery."
- Challenging patient 3: "I did these things but it didn't help at all. It's just a drop in the bucket. And now [my therapist] and family are going to expect me to do more and more."

As illustrated above, patients' cognitions can facilitate or hinder their ability or willingness to make even small changes in their behavior. And having made changes, their thoughts influence whether or not they will make further changes. *When patients are not functioning well, changing what they do from day to day is an essential part of getting better.* For many patients, especially those who are depressed, this means becoming more active, decreasing their avoidance, and increasing their opportunities to experience mastery and pleasure. (For patients who are trying to fulfill too many responsibilities, the therapist's goal would be different, of course: limiting nonessential tasks and building in more opportunities for rest and relaxation—and pleasure).

"Easy" patients generally believe that focusing on problem solving is useful, that they are capable enough to make changes, and that making changes will make them feel better and allow them to have a better life. Patients with challenging problems, on the other hand, may have a number of dysfunctional cognitions. They may believe that their problems are insoluble or that they are incapable of solving their problems; that focusing on problem solving will make them feel worse, not better; that their therapist will hurt them in some way if they reveal their problems; that agreeing to make changes means that they are weak or inferior; or that actually making changes between sessions will diminish them or make them worse off in some way. These same cognitions may have also been activated during and interfered with initial goal setting (see Chapter 7).

Some of these patients, nevertheless, can modify their beliefs through standard techniques and progress well. At the other extreme are patients who need extensive belief modification before they are willing to make any significant change.

USING AND VARYING STANDARD STRATEGIES TO FACILITATE PROBLEM SOLVING

Difficulties in getting patients to focus on problem solving and making changes for homework may be due to patients' dysfunctional beliefs and coping strategies. However, many problems are related to difficulties *therapists* have in employing and varying strategies to facilitate collaborative problem solving. These strategies, described below, include helping patients focus on a problem, motivating patients through psychoeducation, making a connection between solving individual problems and achieving goals, breaking down problems into manageable parts, helping patients assess their degree of control, and changing course when problem solving is not working.

Helping Patients Focus on a Problem

A common difficulty in getting a patient to do problem solving arises when patients *jump from one problem to the next* in session. The usual strategy is for the therapist to interrupt and make the patient conscious of the change (then collaboratively decide which problems to focus on):

> ■ "Sorry to interrupt, but I just wanted to make sure what we should talk about. We started with [how lonely you feel at night] but now we've changed to [dealing with your ex-husband]—which do you think is more important right now?"

If patients do not have dysfunctional cognitions about focusing on a problem, they are likely to respond well to their therapist's collaborative attempt to direct the session productively.

A second common difficulty arises when a patient's *level of distress is too high* at the moment to focus on solving a problem. Roberta was so upset about an argument with a coworker that she could not adopt a problem-solving frame of mind. The therapist empathized, then gave the patient a choice:

> ■ "I'm sorry you're feeling so distressed—and it seems like the more you talk about [how Douglas affected you], the worse you feel. (*pause*) Do you think it might be better to talk about [a lesser problem] now and get back to Douglas later?"

Motivating Patients through Psychoeducation

Some patients need additional psychoeducation before they are willing to engage in problem solving. It is important to tell patients that coming to treatment by itself will not alleviate their suffering and help them feel better. They need to make small changes in their thinking and behavior on a daily basis.

Patients may balk at discussing how they can become more active, for example, and need the therapist to explain that engaging in activities that have the potential to increase their pleasure and mastery are important if they are to feel better. The therapist may need to help them recognize that *waiting* until they feel better to engage in these kinds of activities has not worked for them—after all they are still symptomatic. Some patients believe that they have to feel motivated *before* they take action. The therapist can help them recognize that they will probably feel more motivated *after* they have started the activity.

When patients believe that they will not have enough energy to carry through with a task, therapists can provide an analogy to making a fire. It does take a certain amount of energy to collect the wood and arrange it properly. But it takes relatively little energy to light the match and throw on another log from time to time. Likewise it takes a certain amount of mental (and sometimes physical) energy to start a task, but once they have started, patients may well find it is easier to continue.

Therapist self-disclosure or a review of the patient's own experience can also help demonstrate that the most difficult period is often just before starting a task (and perhaps for the next minute or two). This is particularly true if the patient is struggling with making the decision of whether or not to start the task.

Another helpful example is to ask patients what they now do automatically, without thinking about how motivated they are or about how much they want to do an activity—for example, brushing their teeth. They do not struggle with the decision; they take it for granted that they will do it. It is important for them to put other activities vital to their recovery in the same "no-choice" category.

Making a Connection between Solving Individual Problems and Achieving Goals

Some patients need to be reminded about a goal they have set for themselves and that they strongly desire before they can fully engage in discussing a problem from the agenda, as mentioned in the previous chapter. Before discussing a problem Kyle had put on the agenda (an argument he had had with his supervisor), his therapist checked to see how important it was to him at the moment to reach his goal of improving his situation at work. Cathy, for example, was not motivated to try to solve her problem of organizing herself at home (paying bills, balancing her checkbook, doing errands) until her therapist helped her see the connection between these activities and her goal—which she strongly desired—of moving out of her parents' house. It was further motivating when her therapist had her visualize walking into her new place, feeling proud and pleased.

Breaking Down Problems into Manageable Parts

Patients often believe that a problem is insoluble because they perceive it as overwhelming. Sonia, a schizoaffective patient, was feeling completely overwhelmed about straightening up the house, so she waited in a chair for hours, hoping that God would tell her what to do. After her therapist helped her to see that God would probably want her to be productive instead of passive, she agreed to make the decision on a practical basis. She and her therapist discussed three tasks that had to be done daily: making her bed, straightening up her bedroom, and doing dishes. She agreed to choose whichever one seemed easiest at the moment. Engaging in the first task usually deactivated her helplessness schema and she was able to continue with other tasks that were not even on the list.

When patients get distressed about working on small aspects of a problem, therapists need to help them see that the way to get better is to make small changes every day, that small changes add up to big changes, and that small changes help strengthen the patient to be able to make other significant changes in the future.

Helping Patients Assess the Degree of Control They Have over a Problem

Some patients believe that problem solving will not help because they perceive that they have no control over a problem. Lily was quite fearful that she would lose her job; she felt quite helpless, out of control, and at the mercy of her critical supervisor. After collecting more data about the situation, it was apparent to the therapist that Lily was probably *not* in imminent danger of being fired, but that she probably did display some maladaptive behaviors at work. When they discussed what Lily could do to make it more likely that she could keep her job *and* what she could do to lose her job, she started to feel more in control—and then was able to act more functionally at work. She kept a running record which she added to in session and at home.

Things I Can Do to Keep My Job	Things I Can Do to Lose My Job
• Keep appointment with [psychiatrist] to see if meds should be changed. • Keep taking medication. • Get to bed between 11 and 11:30. • Smile more at work, keep head up even if I don't feel like it. • Read therapy notes. • Talk more to supervisor. • Keep getting to work on time.	• Don't go to see psychiatrist. • Don't take meds. • Go to bed after 1 a.m. • Isolate at work, don't make eye contact with anyone, don't smile, keep head down. • Don't read therapy notes. • Keep telling myself I'm going to get fired. • Avoid supervisor altogether. • Get to work late.

At the bottom of the paper (a copy of which Lily took home to read everyday), she wrote her conclusion:

When I think there's nothing I can do to keep my job
I probably have more control over keeping my job than I think. I can make it more likely by doing the left-side behaviors and avoiding the right-side behaviors. I really want to keep my job and it's worth doing these things even if I feel uncomfortable or put out.

Changing Course When Problem Solving Is Not Working

Sometimes therapists find they are not making any headway on a particular problem and need to make a collaborative agreement to change the focus of discussion or change the topic.

Case Example

Olivia, a patient with schizoaffective disorder periodically became suspicious of people when she was more depressed. When she was euthymic, however, she did not suspect others of malicious motives, and her therapist suspected that her negative view of her coworkers when she was depressed was distorted.

The first time her therapist tried to discuss her paranoid thoughts about others, Olivia was too symptomatic to evaluate her cognitions. The therapist suggested that they change the focus of their discussion. They started to examine how Olivia could cope at work, even if people were being critical of her. They agreed that it would be best if she could put on a good face and respond to them neutrally. Then they talked about the *meaning* of their criticism—that it would lead to her losing her job—and decatastrophized her fear. Her homework assignment, in addition to reading therapy notes, was to try to act naturally and to notice how her coworkers responded to her: the expressions on their faces, their body language, their words and tone of voice.

When Olivia was less depressed and no longer believed her coworkers were malicious, her therapist returned to the original problem and prepared her for the possibility that she might erroneously conclude that her coworkers had negative intentions the next time she became depressed.

USING AND VARYING STANDARD STRATEGIES TO FACILITATE HOMEWORK COMPLETION

Patients with challenging problems are notorious for having difficulty following through with homework assignments. The strategies described below are often effective *unless* the patient holds interfering beliefs (described toward the end of this chapter). Therapists should design homework carefully, ascertain how likely patients are to follow through with the assignment, elicit and address predicted obstacles and interfering cognitions, help patients develop realistic expectations for how much homework will help, address negative thoughts after doing homework, review the assignment at the next session, and, when applicable, conceptualize why patients had difficulty doing the assignment.

Design Homework Carefully

Patients are far more likely to complete homework assignments when the therapist:

- Tailors homework to the individual.
- Provides a rationale.
- Sets the assignment collaboratively.
- Asks the patient to start the assignment in session (when applicable).
- Makes sure the assignment is written down.
- Helps set up reminder systems.
- Anticipates potential problems.

As described below, therapists may also need to suggest easier rather than harder assignments, specify how often and how long patients should spend on each assignment, use alternate terms for "homework," and label assignments as experiments.

Suggest "Easy" Assignments

Therapists who have patients with challenging problems need to be especially cautious in devising homework, and usually need to ensure that the assignments will be relatively easy for the patient to do. Therapists often vastly underestimate the difficulty either of the task itself or of patients' ability to motivate and organize themselves enough to do the task. Early in therapy, for example, patients with challenging problems are far more likely to be able to respond effectively to their thoughts if they read therapy notes (created in the therapy session) rather than trying to complete Dysfunctional Thought Records (J. Beck, 2005). Many patients also lack important prerequisite skills, such as being organized and using their time effectively. They may need instruction in those skills or homework assignments may need to be modified.

Specify the Frequency and Duration of the Assignment

Patients with challenging problems often overestimate the difficulty of an assignment and the time and energy it will take to carry it out. When applicable, it is helpful for therapists to give patients a range of frequency and duration for each assignment: "Do you think you could read these therapy notes twice a day, say, at breakfast and at dinner time? I think it'll take you less than a minute." "How many times this week do you think you could call [specific friends and family members]? Two or three times?"

Change the Label "Homework"

It is also helpful to determine the label patients would like to give to homework. Terms such as "self-help assignment," "wellness plan," "take-out therapy," or "therapy-to-go" are sometimes more palatable to the patient.

Formulate Assignments as Experiments

It is desirable to set up relevant homework assignments as experiments. Research has shown that depressed patients generally feel better when they get more active (Hopko, Le Juez, Ruggiero, & Eifert, 2003). "Would you be willing to do an experiment this week? We can figure out some activities for you to do—then you can see what effect doing them has on how you feel."

Framing behavior change as an experiment helps therapists maintain credibility if patients do not experience a positive affect shift. If this is the case, therapists can, at the next session, elicit the thoughts that interfered with the patient's ability to obtain a sense of pleasure or mastery from engaging in the activities. They can also explain that perhaps patients need a broader set of interventions over a longer period of time before they experience a shift in mood.

Determine the Likelihood That Patients Will Do the Assignment

Having set a homework assignment, perhaps the single most useful question for therapists to ask is:

> ■ "How likely are you to [do this assignment]?"

Patients who respond "90–100%" or "very likely" usually complete the assignment (unless they are overly optimistic or want to avoid further discussion). Patients who say "80%" or "Likely, I guess" usually do part of the assignment, often just to please the therapist. Patients who say "50%" or "I'm not sure" are highly unlikely to do the assignment. Having received a response that is less than 90%, the therapist needs to investigate practical impediments and cognitions that are likely to interfere—or to change the assignment so that the patient is overwhelmingly likely to do it. If a patient is not likely to carry out a behavioral task (e.g., calling a friend), it is preferable to make the task optional or to change the task (e.g., think about calling a friend, think about what I could say; see what thoughts get in the way of calling him/her).

Elicit and Respond in Advance to Interfering Cognitions

Asking patients to focus on their emotions and thoughts as they imagine doing a homework assignment can often elicit interfering cognitions. After discussing an adaptive response, and then asking the patient to summarize the discussion, the patient (or therapist) should write down his/her conclusions. (Alternatively, the patient or therapist could audiotape the summary at the time or at the end of the session.) For example:

Automatic thought: I don't feel like getting out of bed.

Response: It's true I don't feel like getting out of bed, but I also don't want to keep feeling this depressed. I need to see what happens if I do get out of bed and get my day started.

Automatic thought: Doing these things won't help.

Response: I haven't gotten better by not doing these things and I don't have a crystal ball. I may actually feel better by doing them.

Automatic thought: Doing this is just a drop in the bucket.

Response: The only way I'm going to get better is by doing small things every day. Over time, these small things will add up to big things.

Automatic thought: I'm not getting better, so why do these things?

Response: My depression won't go away overnight. Don't expect to feel great changes right away. The important thing is to keep doing productive things.

Automatic thought: If I get better, I won't have any reason to stay home.

Response: When I get better, I'll have the *choice* about whether to stay home or not. Now I'm depressed and don't have any choices.

Automatic thought: I'm too tired or stressed to do this.

Response: It will only take 10 minutes. I can do anything for 10 minutes. Not doing it makes me feel like I'm too helpless to get better. It's important to prove to myself that I can do things. Paying too much attention to my energy level will keep me stuck where I am now.

> **Automatic thought:** It's okay if I don't do this [or I'll do it later].
>
> **Response:** It's important to do this every time. It's *not* okay to postpone it. Every time I do something I don't want to do, I strengthen a healthy muscle that will lead me to my goals. Every time I don't, I strengthen my procrastination muscle that leads me away from reaching my goals.

> **Automatic thought:** It's unfair that I have to do this.
>
> **Response:** It's more unfair to myself to keep feeling so depressed everyday.

Help Patients Develop Realistic Expectations for How Much Homework Is Likely to Help

Some patients with challenging problems require significant intervention before they start to notice a change in their mood. It is important that they have a realistic expectation; otherwise, they may become quite hopeless and terminate therapy prematurely. The goal of homework for these patients, therefore, is not to feel better *immediately*, but instead to build skills (e.g., activity scheduling or responding to negative cognitions) and create positive experiences that will culminate over time in an improvement in mood. It is helpful for these patients to write down their homework assignment with its rationale. For example:

> Go for at least a 5-minute walk everyday even if it doesn't make me feel better because it's a first step in taking control of my depression.

It is also important for these patients to give themselves credit every time they do a homework assignment and to recognize that doing so is incrementally moving them toward their goal. Therapy notes can help remind them to do so.

> Every time I do my therapy homework—or any productive task—remind myself that I deserve credit, especially if I don't see an immediate payoff.

Address Negative Thoughts after Doing Homework

Instead of giving themselves credit, however, some patients unwittingly undermine their progress with negative thinking after completing a homework assignment. If a patient does not feel better after doing a potentially rewarding assignment, the therapist should probe for interfering thoughts that arose during the assignment and afterwards and help patients devise adaptive responses that they can read after doing their homework. The following examples are drawn from the three challenging patients described at the beginning of this chapter.

Automatic thought: I did these things, but I didn't do them very well and now I'm exhausted. Therapy isn't helping. I'll never feel better.

Response: I deserve credit for just doing these things. After all, I hadn't been doing them before I started therapy. It will take time for me to feel better. I wish these things would make me feel better immediately, but that's unrealistic. I just need to keep doing them and keep going to treatment.

Automatic thought: I did all these things but I hated doing them. It's not fair that I should have to spend my life in drudgery.

Response: Doing these things does feel like drudgery, especially because I'm depressed and have less energy. They will be a little easier to do when I get less depressed. And I need to work in therapy to schedule positive things in my life, too, and create a better balance.

Automatic thought: I did these things but it didn't help at all. It's just a drop in the bucket. And now [my therapist] and family are going to expect me to do more and more.

Response: It was important to do these things, even though I didn't feel better immediately. Eventually, when I make enough changes, I will feel better. [My therapist] wants me to tell her if I think she expects too much from me. And if Susie and the kids start expecting too much, I can tell them I need more time.

Review the Assignment at the Next Session

As described in the previous chapter, it is essential to review homework assignments at the next session. Doing so emphasizes the importance of homework and motivates patients to keep doing it. It also gives the therapist an opportunity to collect needed data, to reinforce what the patient has learned from the assignment, and to assess whether it would be desirable for the patient to continue the assignment in the coming week.

Conceptualize the Difficulty When Patients Do Not Do the Assignment

First it is important to determine whether there was a practical obstacle that interfered with the patient's ability to do homework—for example, the patient did not understand what to do, became ill, or had a genuine lack of opportunity. If not, therapists should assess whether they themselves followed the guidelines above. Finally, therapists may need to ask patients to remember a specific time during which they thought about doing a homework assignment but did not follow through. Imagining the incident as if it is happening right now allows the patient to have greater access to his/her interfering thoughts. Responding to these cognitions, as described below, will be key in ensuring that patients will complete their therapy homework in the future.

DYSFUNCTIONAL BELIEFS THAT INTERFERE WITH PROBLEM SOLVING AND DOING HOMEWORK

Despite reasonable preparation, some patients still refrain from focusing on solving problems and doing homework. Often their highly ingrained and rigid beliefs interfere. This section describes how to elicit and modify these beliefs.

Identifying Key Beliefs

There are several ways to uncover beliefs that interfere with problem solving or doing homework: eliciting the conditional assumption, identifying disadvantages, and using a checklist.

Eliciting the Conditional Assumption

The therapist can provide part of a conditional assumption and ask the patient for its meaning or for a feared outcome:

> ■ "If you were to [focus more deeply on this problem/solve this problem/go ahead and do homework], what would that mean?"
> ■ "What might that lead to?"
> ■ "What might be bad about that?"

Eliciting Disadvantages

Another way to collect the same kind of information is to find out from the patient's point of view why solving the problem or doing homework might be disadvantageous:

> ■ "It seems to me as if there could be some advantages to trying to solve this problem, but I'm guessing that there are some *disadvantages*, too. (*pause*) What might the disadvantages be?"

If the patient is not forthcoming, the therapist can try hypothesizing about and normalizing their concerns:

> ■ "Some people don't want to talk about [improving things with their family] because it makes them feel [as if they themselves did something wrong . . . or they feel that solving the problem will let their family off the hook]. . . . Does it seem like that to you?"

Using a Checklist

Therapists can also ask patients to fill the out checklist, "Possible Reasons For Not Doing Self-Help Assignments" (Beck, Rush, Shaw, & Emery, 1979). Some patients may be more willing to check off items on the form than to verbalize their concerns. They can complete the form in session or at home when they find themselves procrastinating on a homework assignment.

Typical Beliefs

Typical interfering beliefs are often related to the meaning patients put to:

- The *process* of therapy
- Their *ability* to be *successful* with therapy
- The *consequences of becoming well*

Typical beliefs in these three categories are described below.

Beliefs about the Process of Therapy

These beliefs are related to patients' perception of being harmed by the process, either because of their internal turmoil or because of the therapist's behavior. One such example was presented in Chapter 5: the patient Mandy who feared her therapist would hurt her if she revealed the abuse she had experienced as a child. Other examples include:

"If I Talk about My Problem, I'll Get So Overwhelmed [with Negative Emotion], I'll Fall Apart."

Before Monica began therapy, her only coping strategy when distressed had been to avoid or leave situations or to distract herself. In session, she used a variety of maneuvers to try to keep a lid on her emotions. She often changed topics, went off on tangents, denied having negative emotions, tried to keep discussions of problems superficial, and agreed with what her therapist said without reflection. Between sessions, Monica failed to do homework. Recognizing a pattern, her therapist asked her what it meant to her to focus more intently on a problem and try to solve it. She revealed a dysfunctional belief about experiencing negative emotion that her therapist then was able to help her evaluate and respond to.

Monica came to realize that while she had had literally hundreds of experiences of feeling highly distressed, she had broken down and needed to be hospitalized only twice. And even then, she had ultimately recovered. Her therapist helped her see how she was different (stronger) now, how she was learning tools in therapy to manage her distress better, and how she was not now experiencing the kind of highly provocative and distressing precipitants that had previously culminated in hospitalization. After several experiences in which she was significantly upset at the beginning of a therapy session but felt somewhat better by the end, she was more willing to focus on problems. She began to see that she could do things to alleviate her distress or at least tolerate it.

Additional strategies to modify this assumption are described in detail in Chapter 12.

"If I Let My Therapist Direct the Session, It Means She's Strong and Superior and I'm Weak and Inferior."

Beliefs such as these indicate a problem in the therapeutic relationship (see Chapters 4 and 5). Sean tried to control his therapy sessions. Whenever his therapist became directive, he kept talking and did not let her interrupt to steer him toward problem solving. He also put her down for suggesting homework assignments: "[Monitoring my moods] won't help at all. I feel lousy all the time. I don't need to keep a record to tell you that!" What really helped was when his therapist, having identified this belief, discussed the bind she was in.

THERAPIST: You know, I've been noticing something. Can you tell me whether you think I'm on target with this? (*taking responsibility*) I think I annoy you whenever I interrupt, or ask questions, or focus on solving a problem. Is that right?

SEAN: Well, yeah.

THERAPIST: It's really important to me that I make this therapy right for you. Can you tell me what it means to you when I interrupt or make a suggestion? What's bad about that?

SEAN: You're just like my old therapist. He was always trying to tell me what to do.

THERAPIST: So when I ask you for details about the argument you had with your son-in-law, for example, it feels like I'm telling you what to do?

SEAN: Yeah, or you're *going* to tell me what to do.

THERAPIST: And if I did tell you what to do, what would be so bad about that?

SEAN: (*irritably*) I don't know. It's like you have all the answers. Like I'm this stupid loser.

THERAPIST: Well, no wonder my questions irritate you. (*pause*) What do you think we can do about this?

SEAN: *I* don't know.

THERAPIST: Well, let me ask you this. Do you think I'm sincere in wanting to help you?

SEAN: (*Thinks.*) Yeah, I guess so.

THERAPIST: Do you think I deliberately want you to feel like that?

SEAN: (*Thinks.*) No, I guess not.

THERAPIST: How do you know that?

SEAN: (*Sighs.*) I guess if you really wanted to, you could put me down. You could act all high and mighty like my first therapist. I fired him, you know.

THERAPIST: Well, I'm glad you don't put me in the same category with him. (*pause*) Now, back to how I can help you if what I say makes you feel like a loser.

SEAN: I don't know. (*pause*) Can I think about it?

THERAPIST: Absolutely. Maybe we can both think about it this week.

SEAN: Okay.

At their next session, the therapist and the patient decided that putting a note saying "Different Category" on the table between the two of them would, throughout the session, remind Sean that perhaps the therapist had benign intentions toward him and would remind the therapist to avoid sounding too bossy or pedantic. They also discussed many other ideas to counter the patient's dysfunctional belief, for example, that a person was smart, not stupid, for allowing someone competent to advise him, much as CEOs of companies or leaders in government are smart to listen to aides with special expertise.

"If I Do What My Therapist Wants Me to Do, It Means She's Controlling Me."

Claire displayed passive–aggressive beliefs and behavioral strategies. She had a knee-jerk reaction, automatically refuting what others (including her therapist) said and refusing to do what others asked. A key intervention involved helping her view her automatic reaction as undesirable—one that indicated that other people were still "pulling her strings," controlling her emotions and behavior. She could "cut the strings" by recognizing when she was having an automatic "opposite reaction," and then reflect on the question: "What is in my long-term best interest to say or do?" Her therapist also was able to get Claire to agree that if saying or doing something benefited someone else, that was okay, as long as it also benefited Claire.

"I Don't Care If I Get Better [So What's the Point of Engaging in Therapy/Doing Homework]."

When patients are quite hopeless, they sometimes have the automatic thought "I don't care." Harriet, a bipolar patient, frequently had this thought when she was more severely depressed and therefore allowed herself to stay in bed, call in sick to work, and generally withdraw from activities and people. Having identified this idea, her therapist helped her evaluate this thought. They devised the following therapy notes:

Response to "I don't care"

It may be true that I don't care right at this moment. But I know from past experience that I *will* care in the future. I always do. I can let this idea defeat me or I can go back to my antidepression plan right now and probably feel better and care again sooner.

At another session they added to the response above to make it more robust:

Not caring is a passing phase. I don't have to pay too much attention to whether I care or not. The important thing is to keep following my plan.

And at another session, they again added to the notes:

It's okay if I don't care, I don't *have* to care to do things.

Beliefs about Helplessness or Failure

Patients express their fears or concerns in different ways:

- "I can't make changes."
- "I'm too helpless."
- "I have no control."
- "My problems are insoluble."
- "I can only get better if my medication works [or someone or something external to me changes]."

The techniques described in the next chapter, such as straightforward Socratic questioning, can help patients shift their perspective on the likelihood of failure. In addition, it is important for therapists to formulate with patients a concrete plan to get better and to help them develop realistic images in which they see themselves acting functionally, solving problems, and feeling better. Also, doing behavioral experiments often demonstrates to them that their beliefs are inaccurate. Case examples of these negative beliefs appear below.

"If I Try to Solve this Problem or Do This Homework Assignment, I'll Fail Because I'm Too Incompetent."

Grace not only had a lifelong belief that she was helpless and incompetent, she had a pervasive coping strategy of procrastination and avoidance. At some level, she thought it was better to live with a problem, even though it led to significant distress. Although such avoidance inevitably led to failure, she could at least say to herself, "I failed because I didn't try," which was less painful than the alternative: "I failed because I'm incompetent." In the short run, this difficulty arose when Grace failed to bring up important problems in therapy and to do therapy homework. Her therapist had to help her modify her belief about incompetence before she was willing to solve problems and do homework.

"I Don't Have Any Control Over My Mood."

These patients often fail to do homework because they do not think it will make any difference in how they feel: "No matter what I try, nothing works. I always feel bad." An important assignment is for patients to monitor their moods to determine whether they do experience any mood fluctuations based on what they are doing and what they are thinking. To get patients to see that they do have at least some control over their mood, it is also helpful for some patients to keep a running list of ways they can make themselves feel worse and ways they can themselves feel better. Larry, for example, was able to mobilize himself after reading a card that reminded him that he usually felt better when he got up right away, took a shower, had breakfast, and took the dog out for a walk—and worse when he stayed in bed late, did not get dressed for hours, and spent most of his time watching television.

"Nothing Will Make a Difference."

In the following transcript, Ellen, a patient with chronic treatment-resistant depression, comes to her fourth therapy session feeling very hopeless. The therapist initially tries to set an agenda with her, but Ellen's hopelessness interferes.

THERAPIST: So what problem do you want to want to work on today?

ELLEN: Oh, I don't know. (*pause*) It's so hopeless.

THERAPIST: So one problem we could work on is your feeling of hopelessness? Do you think we should also talk about work, or your husband?

ELLEN: I don't know. (*trying to shift the responsibility to the therapist*) Whatever you think.

THERAPIST: (*trying to shift the responsibility back to Ellen*) Actually, I'm not sure what would make the biggest difference to you.

ELLEN: It doesn't matter. I don't think anything will make a difference.

THERAPIST: Well, that sounds like an important thought for us to work on when we get to hopelessness.

The therapist continues with the bridge between sessions and the patient agrees to put "problem with husband" on the agenda as well. Next, they begin discussing the initial agenda item of hopelessness.

THERAPIST: Is it okay if we start with your thought "Nothing will make a difference"?

ELLEN: Yeah.

THERAPIST: How much do you believe *right now*—(*emphasizing the collaborative nature of working together*) that working on a problem *with me*—let's say, [mentioning a goal patient might find desirable], or helping you schedule your life better, adding in more enjoyable activities—won't make a difference?

ELLEN: (*changing her tune a little*) Well, it might make a little difference but in the scheme of things . . . it won't matter much.

THERAPIST: (*agreeing with part of what Ellen has said*) Well, the truth of it is, you're *partially* right. Scheduling activities, if that's *all* we do together, won't make much of a difference. Scheduling activities will *only* work if it's part of a *larger* antidepression package . . . . We've talked about this before—learning to answer back your depressed thinking, solving the problems with your husband, figuring out how to be more comfortable at work. (*pause*) It's going to take *all* these things together to make a lasting difference.

ELLEN: (*Looks away.*)

THERAPIST: Ellen, is there a disadvantage to doing these things to try to get over your depression?

ELLEN: It just feels like too much.

THERAPIST: (*partially agreeing with patient*) You're right. It *is* too much ... *if* you think you have to do *everything* at once. (*pause*) What do you think? Are you better off this week taking some *small* steps like going to the movies or having coffee with your friend Bonnie . . . or *not* doing those things?

ELLEN: Doing those things, I guess. (*Thinks.*) But going for walks or going to the movies isn't going to suddenly make me feel better.

THERAPIST: No, you're right. So if you decide to do those things you'll have to remind yourself *not* to expect to feel much different in the short run—but instead, give yourself credit for doing things now that will have a payoff later on.

ELLEN: Hmmmn.

THERAPIST: Ellen, can you summarize for me what we've just talked about?

ELLEN: (*Sighs.*) Well, you're trying to convince me that I should do small things because it'll have a payoff later.

THERAPIST: And what do you think?

ELLEN: I guess that could be right.

THERAPIST: Would you be willing to try some things this week even though you're not very hopeful?

ELLEN: I guess so.

THERAPIST: Are you sure? Or are there other ways you think will help more?

ELLEN: No, I guess not. (*Thinks.*) Well, sure, if my husband suddenly started being nice to me.

THERAPIST: That *would* be great. Is it likely?

ELLEN: (*glumly*) No.

THERAPIST: So if you want to feel better, I suppose it's up to *you* to make changes in your life: to stay home on the couch or get up and take a walk. To sit in front of the TV or call someone to go to a movie with you.

ELLEN: (*pause*) Yeah.

THERAPIST: Ready to commit to something for homework?

ELLEN: Yeah.

THERAPIST: Well, why don't we brainstorm about some possibilities—then we can figure out whether you want to commit to them or (*giving her an out so she will not feel coerced*) whether you should make them optional again this week.

Following this discussion, Ellen commits to doing several small activities. She and her therapist compose alternative responses which she writes down on cards to read everyday. These cards provide responses to dysfunctional thoughts Ellen predicts she might have before and after doing an activity. Then the therapist probes to see whether there might be other unspoken disadvantages to Ellen's changing: fears of getting her hopes up, then having them dashed; concerns about raised expectations of her; a negative impact on her relationship with her husband; or any special (negative) meanings to getting better. There seemed to be none.

Ellen was able to carry out some of the homework assignments and started to feel less helpless and hopeless, which then made it easier for her to continue working in session and between sessions.

As the above vignette illustrates, some patients believe that there is nothing they can do that will matter or make a difference. However, it may be argued that it is a physical reality that *everything* the patient does will have some impact on what happens next in his or her life, and thus is inherently important (McCullough, 2000).

"I Need [a 'Magic Bullet']."

Samantha did not believe she could help herself feel better. She was always looking for a "magic bullet": a new therapy, a new medication, a new job, a new boyfriend. She had become increasingly discouraged and hopeless. By the time she started cognitive therapy (her sixth attempt at psychotherapy in 15 years), she still expected her therapist to magically "fix" her; she didn't believe that she could "fix" herself. In fact she spent long periods every day fantasizing that she was being rescued: by a new boyfriend ("a knight in shining armor"), by a beneficent boss who recognized how special she was, by a therapist. Her therapist helped Samantha recognize that fantasizing helped her feel better momentarily but that she always felt worse by the end of the day when she recognized how little she had accomplished and how poorly she felt. Her therapist empathized with her and gave her permission to express her disappointment. "I wish I *could* make you feel all better right now—but that's just not possible. It must be disappointing to you that I can't." Later they discussed what the therapist *could* do: "Help *you* help *yourself* to feel better." After a significant discussion, they devised the following response:

When I fantasize about being saved

The evidence is that if I wait for someone to save me, I'll continue to feel miserable. With [my therapist's help], I can "save" myself. That's the only way I'm going to feel better. The fantasy of a savior makes me feel better, but only momentarily, and then I feel worse.

Beliefs about Getting Better or Becoming Well

These negative beliefs may relate to an immediate negative outcome patients perceive or to the long-term outcome of recovering from their disorder.

"If I Discover Ways to Solve This Problem, It Will Show That I've Been Wrong [Which Is Intolerable to Me]."

Hank did not want to talk about how to make his day at work more tolerable because at some level he knew that he bore some of the responsibility for problems there. He tried to speak at length about how unfairly others treated him and avoided the therapist's questions when she tried to get a better idea of what had happened, what Hank had said and done. The following transcript illustrates a key intervention:

THERAPIST: (*empathically*) Obviously your coworkers said and did some hurtful things. No wonder you're so upset! To be able to help you with this, I need to know what you said and did, too. Is there something bad about talking about that?

HANK: I don't know what you mean.

THERAPIST: (*normalizing*) Oh, some patients find it hard to talk about what *they* did, especially if they're not proud of it, or if they think it contributed to the problem—or if they think I'll blame them. (*pause*) I was wondering, is it hard for you?

"If I Find a Solution to This Problem, It Means I've Suffered Needlessly."

Kimberly had suffered for many years as her elderly father's caretaker. When her therapist suggested some straightforward solutions, such as leaving the room when he yelled at her, setting limits with him, rewarding him for positive behavior, and getting respite care from other members of the family and from social services, Kimberly disparaged every idea. It was too painful for her to admit that she might have been able to solve some of her difficulties with her father years earlier. She was able to acknowledge that this was the case, however, when her therapist hypothesized about this possibility ("Kimberly, I wonder if it's difficult for you to consider that you might have the power to make things better. For example, would it be bad for you to find out that you could have made things better a while ago?").

Patients may experience an existential crisis when they recognize that they have spent precious time in needless, self-imposed suffering (Yalom, 1980). One way to soften the blow is to consider the possibility that the patient is only now at a stage of psychological development where he or she can make the leap from self-perceived victim to self-efficacious individual. Thus, previous time (and perhaps previous years in therapy) may not be a waste after all—to the contrary—they may be natural precursors to the patient's current state of mind and improved future possibilities.

"If I Get My Hopes Up, I'll Get Terribly Disappointed."

Although it made sense to Vince to solve problems in session and to do homework, he resisted doing so because he was afraid that solving his initial problems would make him feel hopeful—and that he would feel even *worse* when, he predicted, he was unable to recover fully. His thera-

pist helped Vince see that if his hopes were not fulfilled, he would probably feel only marginally worse than he did at the present. On the other
hand, if he tried new behaviors, there probably would be substantial
reward, worth the risk of possible disappointment.

"If I Focus on Solving a Problem and Agree to Do Homework, I'll Have to Do Things I Don't Want to Do."

Alaina spent most of several therapy sessions trying to convince her
therapist how terrible she felt and how bad her life was. Every time her
therapist asked if she wanted to try to solve one of her problems, Alaina
answered with a "Yes, but" statement: "Yes, but you see, even if I talk to
my mother about this, it won't do any good because she . . . "; "Yes, but I
know if I try to get out of bed earlier, I'll be so exhausted, I'll just climb
right back in and then . . . ." Her therapist conceptualized that Alaina's
difficulties had less to do with a belief that she was helpless and more to
do with an unwillingness to change. He hypothesized aloud:

THERAPIST: So, Alaina, it sounds as if you have the idea "No matter what I
     do, it won't work."

ALAINA: Yeah, maybe.

THERAPIST: Or "I can't get myself to do it."

ALAINA: I guess.

THERAPIST: Alaina, I'm wondering, how much do you think it's also "I
     don't *want* to do it?"

ALAINA: (*pause*) I don't know.

THERAPIST: Well, how much do you *want* to get out of bed and start your
     day earlier?

ALAINA: Not much, I guess.

THERAPIST: And how much do you *want* to make things better with your
     mom?

ALAINA: That witch. (*pause*) I don't, I guess.

THERAPIST: Maybe we need to talk about what you *do* want, then, and how
     you see yourself getting it.

Before Alaina was willing to put significant effort toward solving her
problems and assume more responsibilities in her life, her therapist had
to do several things: review her goals and establish that Alaina really did
not want to continue her unsatisfying lifestyle and *did* want to lead a more
functional life; carefully elicit and reframe the disadvantages of solving
problems and getting better; reduce Alaina's anger toward her mother;
address Alaina's anxious predictions about her capability of meeting spe-

cific challenges (especially returning to work); and help Alaina create a positive, realistic, concrete image of a typical day 6 months in the future when she no longer felt as depressed.

Other patients are not immediately concerned with having to do things they do not want to do, but they fear that *if* they start doing these things, they will *eventually* have to do other things that are unpalatable to them. Tara feared that once she appeared more functional, her partner would give back to her the many responsibilities he had taken on that formerly had been hers: paying bills, doing the food shopping, preparing meals. Tara recognized that she would have to go back to doing things she did not want to do.

"If I Try to Solve This Problem Productively, I Will Have to Let Others Off the Hook."

Abe believed that he had been badly mistreated by his family of origin for years. He resisted talking about how he could make an upcoming trip home better for himself. The idea of treating his family reasonably felt invalidating to him. He still wanted to punish them for their misdeeds, even at a significant emotional cost to himself.

Abe's therapist had him recall his previous trip home, when he had punished his family by refusing to attend a family reunion, go with them to the zoo, or join in on a family project to organize photographs. He remembered how isolated, unconnected, even rejected he had felt, and how the hurt had persisted for weeks and weeks afterward. His therapist helped him realize that his family members had probably felt minimally hurt compared to Abe. After their discussion, Abe recognized that if he used the same strategy to punish them, he himself would probably end up being punished much more. Abe finally concluded that it was worth it to him to do what he could to reduce his own pain, given that his family would probably not feel very pained in any case.

"If I Focus on How I Need to Change (Stop Punishing) to Get Better, I'll Get Hurt Again."

Amanda, like Abe, wanted to punish someone else. She was quite angry at her husband, who had had a brief affair 2 years earlier, and initially rejected discussing how she herself could make changes to improve the relationship. She had several ideas that interfered with her motivation:

- "He did something horribly wrong and it's not fair to me to work on solving problems instead of punishing him."
- "Punishing him makes me feel more in control, more powerful."
- "If I don't punish him, he could stray and I could get hurt again."

Amanda's therapist had to help her take a different perspective before she was willing to change. They carefully examined the disadvantages of continuing to punish her husband: it kept her all stirred up emotionally; she was providing a poor role model for her children; she was perhaps making it *more* likely that he would indeed stray again; although it made her feel somewhat more powerful, it also made her feel "crummy" to treat him badly. Her therapist had her imagine three scenarios taking place on a typical day a year from the present. He asked her to focus each time on how she felt and on her general sense of well-being. In the first scenario, Amanda imagined herself still treating her husband poorly. In a second scenario, she imagined that they had separated, due to another affair, and that she was coping with the separation well. In the final scenario, she imagined that they had stayed together and that she had been treating him well for the entire year. She finally concluded that it was in her best interest to stop punishing her husband and to try to rebuild a reasonable relationship with him (see Spring, 1996, for more on this subject).

"If I Get Better, I'll Have to Face a Difficult Challenge."

Diane realized that as long as she was highly symptomatic, she had no choice: she needed her husband to support her. If she got better, however, and no longer needed him, she would have to face the fact that her marriage was quite poor and she thought it would mean she would have to make the decision to divorce her husband. Her therapist helped her see that once she got over her chronic panic disorder and agoraphobia, she would have the *choice* of whether to divorce or not; it did not automatically mean that she would *have* to get divorced. He also helped her see that she had no way of knowing at the moment how her relationship with her husband might change if he no longer felt so burdened by her illness.

"If I Get Better, It Means I Lose."

Some patients know they will suffer a monetary loss if they get better. They may no longer be eligible for disability benefits or they may receive a reduced award in a lawsuit for pain and suffering. Others predict they will suffer a different loss. Adam knew he would have to go back to high school full time instead of receiving minimal tutoring at home. Ava was afraid her parents would no longer be emotionally supportive and that her therapist would make her terminate from therapy if she got better. If Linda recovered from her depression, she recognized that she would have to fulfill her role: go back to business as usual—her "life of drudgery" as a homemaker, the mother of two recalcitrant adolescents, and the wife of a husband who was willing to take over household responsibilities only when Linda was unwell.

The therapist had to help these patients focus on the long-term goals they wanted for themselves. She helped them evaluate just how deleterious the loss would be and how they could cope with or make up for the loss. Then he had them imagine a day in the future in which they had reached their goals and were compensating for the loss.

Evan's therapist had to make some additional interventions. Getting better would mean Evan would have to get a job. Getting a job meant that his father and his wife (who continually nagged him to get back to work) would "win" and he would lose. His therapist helped him see how much he was currently losing by *not* working: he was in bad financial straits, his self-esteem was at an all-time low, he had gained weight and was out of shape, he did not have the comradery of his coworkers, he was embarrassed to tell people he was still out of work. She also role-played with Evan how he could tell his wife and father that he was going back to work, emphasizing that he had made this decision for himself (and intimating that it was not because *they* wanted him to).

Some patients are unwilling to make changes until they face unpalatable consequences. Kevin was unwilling to follow through with making even small changes in his day-to-day life. He was spending a great deal of time in bed. His belief was that if he could prove to his father that he was utterly miserable, his father would not make him get a job but instead would fund his studies at the trade school he wanted to attend. A family session did not convince him otherwise. It was not until his father stopped providing him with money—so that he was unable to drive his car, buy himself DVDs and CDs, or go to the movies—that Kevin began to see that his father meant business and he became more willing to make changes. His therapy notes helped remind him of the choices he could make.

When I'm tempted to do nothing

The evidence is that Dad has changed. He probably won't give me money, even if I continue to nag him or yell at him. I can continue to stay in my room and feel miserable *or* I can make the decision to take control of my life. I can start with small things like getting up early everyday, taking a shower, eating properly, going for walks and doing other things that don't cost money until I'm ready to get a job.

"If I Get Better, I Won't Know Who I Am."

Phil's identity was wrapped up in his illness. He couldn't imagine who he would be if he no longer suffered from panic disorder and severe agoraphobia. Patients like Phil, who see themselves and their psychological disorders as inextricably linked, often view the concept of wellness as the great unknown, a frightening notion that can keep them stuck where they are (see Mahoney, 1991). In response to this problem, Phil's therapist used strategies described in Chapter 13 to help patients deal with their anxiety when they first start to question the validity of their core beliefs.

CASE EXAMPLE

Patricia was a 44-year-old married woman with a teenage son. She entered therapy with severe depression (her third episode since childhood), anxiety, and strong passive–aggressive traits. A precipitating factor had been her husband's losing his job (through no fault of his own). At first she was highly anxious about their worsening financial situation. As Patricia became convinced that her husband would not be able to find a job that paid more than minimum wage, she became more and more depressed.

Patricia's functioning had deteriorated significantly. Although she got up every morning to make breakfast for her son and see him off to school, she stayed in bed most of the day, neglecting the upkeep of the house. She did not get up again until he was about to come home. She prepared dinner for the family but crawled back into bed as soon as her husband came home from his part-time job.

In the first few therapy sessions, Patricia agreed to standard homework and, when asked, said she was likely to do it. She returned to subsequent sessions, however, having half-heartedly completed only a small part of it. For example, in the second session she reported that she could recall some of her automatic thoughts from the past week but she had not written any down, nor had she read her therapy notes that reminded her that some of her thoughts might not be true, or not completely true, since she was so depressed. She had not made any of the behavioral changes she had agreed to in the first session.

Her therapist first tried standard techniques, such as breaking tasks down into smaller steps and helping her respond to her automatic thoughts. Initially her thoughts all had a theme of helplessness and, based on their discussion, she and her therapist prepared notes to help her counteract them.

Automatic thought: If I try to do pleasurable activities, I won't feel any better.

Response: Actually, I don't know if I'll feel better or not—and I won't know unless I try. Even if they don't help me feel better in the short run, they may in the long run.

Automatic thought: If I do feel better, it won't last long.

Response: That may be true initially, but I can learn skills to affect my mood for longer periods.

Automatic thought: I can't take care of the house. Even if I try to straighten things up, I won't be able to do it. There's too much to do. Besides, it won't matter, the house will still be messy.

Response: Doing *anything* more around the house than I'm now doing is really a success. I can get the house in order, step by step. I can't do it all at once—but that's *not* the plan anyway.

Automatic thought and image: If only I could hole up some place and not have to do anything, I could get better.

Response: Having no structure, no activities with other people, no reason to get out of bed, no opportunity to accomplish things will probably make me feel worse, not better.

Automatic thought: This therapy isn't for me. I'm not the sort of person who can follow a schedule.

Response: Not following a schedule hasn't made me feel less depressed. I can experiment with trying a schedule for a week or two and see if it makes me feel better or worse.

Responding to these helpless thoughts over the next couple of weeks helped slightly and Patricia began to do just a little more around the house, though she would not try to follow even a minimal schedule. Despite these positive changes, her depression did not budge. In fact, she became somewhat more anxious. A key cognition was:

"If I make changes, my husband will expect more and more of me."

Patricia also reported an unpleasant dream. Someone was insisting that she play with her child's set of dominoes. She had to set the dominoes on end, close to another. This person knocked down the first domino that then set up a chain reaction; all the other dominoes quickly fell, one by one. To Patricia, the dream meant to her that she would have to start making significant changes, and that once she started, she would have no choice but to keep changing.

Patricia's therapist coached her to talk to her husband about having realistic expectations for her. When she failed to do so, he suggested that they invite Patricia's husband in for part of their next session. When she expressed her fear that he would expect her to change back to her old self overnight, he reassured her otherwise. For 2 or 3 weeks, Patricia made some minimal gains. Her anxiety and depression lessened slightly, but then she became more irritable. A key dysfunctional idea was:

"If I do things I don't want to do, it diminishes me."

Upon reviewing her history, it became apparent that Patricia had resisted doing what she did not want to do ever since adolescence. This belief had contributed to her lack of success at jobs she had held before her son was born. At times, however, she had been able to overcome this idea.

For example, she had a very strong sense of the importance of being a good mother to her child, and she had been able, for many years, to get herself to do things that she did not particularly enjoy, but which she knew were essential for her son's well-being. Now that he was older, and she was so depressed, she no longer felt as responsible for doing things that she saw as nonessential. Her therapist was able to help Patricia see at an intellectual level that this idea of diminishment was dysfunctional and inaccurate. It took a long time for her to believe it at an emotional level, though, and she was still struggling with it somewhat when her depression remitted and therapy ended.

Patricia's therapist discussed with her the fact that she had two problems. One, she had real-life responsibilities that felt burdensome, exhausting, never-ending, and unrewarding. To make matters worse, however, she struggled with herself about whether or not to do any given household task. Her therapist tried to get her to see that doing tasks did not diminish her as much as the struggle. After all, she did not believe her sister and her friend Nan were diminished by doing the same tasks.

As Patricia became slightly more functional at home and as bills started piling up, she revealed another important disadvantage to getting better: she would have to get a job. She was enormously reluctant to go back to work and her anxiety and depression worsened significantly as the family's savings continued to dwindle. She could only foresee terrible costs to going to work, including a negative impact on her son and on herself, having to bear the unfairness of having to work, and giving up a strong desire to be rescued. At first she focused on her concern that she would have to neglect her child. Discussing the practical implications of a job, Patricia realized that she would likely return home just an hour after her son usually did and the impact on him would likely be far less than she had predicted.

Then Patricia expressed concerns about the impact on herself, both immediate and longer term effects: "Whatever job I get will be hard. I'll probably hate it. And I'll be exhausted." She had an image of herself (that was partially a memory) behind a sales counter in the late afternoon, feeling incapable, exhausted, and trapped. Her therapist labeled this image as the worst possible outcome, and asked her if she could imagine in detail a realistically better image. At first Patricia resisted trying to create a more positive image. When her therapist asked her what it meant to her to imagine a better future, she replied:

PATRICIA: It won't happen.

THERAPIST: (*hypothesizing*) Are you also concerned that if we paint a better picture, then you might actually have to go out and get a job?

PATRICIA: Yeah, I guess so.

THERAPIST: And what does it mean to you to get a job?

PATRICIA: I'll be trapped. It will be deadly. Once I get a job, I'll have to keep it. I'll have to give up any hope for a happy life.

Her therapist then discussed with her how she could cope if she did get a job that was unbearable and helped her see that she would not be trapped, that she could stick it out for a few days or weeks, in the meantime looking for another job. She could quit the moment she found a better one. They also discussed how *not* having a job was not bringing Patricia happiness either; in fact, she had been growing increasingly despondent and anxious over the past few weeks. Finally, she was willing to imagine what a better job would look like: one that she felt capable of doing, with compatible coworkers and a reasonable boss.

Then Patricia brought up her dread of the long-term impact of getting a job. She could only envision a painful future, a miserable existence of going to work, coming home to a disorderly house, making dinner, cleaning up, going to bed, then waking up and repeating this cycle, for months and years on end. Again her therapist helped her see that she was imagining only the worst possible outcome. They discussed the best possible outcome and the most realistic outcome. Then her therapist had Patricia envision a relatively satisfying day about a year later, when she had been working for several months in a tolerable job, was accustomed to the rhythm of the workday, came home, was glad to see her son, and felt good generally succeeding in her job and helping contribute financially to the family.

Next Patricia reported her fears that she would not be able to be competent in whatever job she got. She had a nightmare that was reminiscent of a childhood struggle she had not previously reported. In the sixth grade, she was required to take a foreign language. She struggled mightily with this subject, and, worse, struggled publicly when she was required to speak dialogue aloud. She had felt extremely embarrassed and had refused to ask the teacher for help. Her therapist conceptualized that this *new* "trauma" (needing to get a job) was perhaps reactivating her feelings of being trapped, helpless, unable to solve her problem. He helped her recognize that these feelings (actually beliefs) were not particularly applicable in the present time. Patricia did not have to take a job that was far beyond her skills, she could try to solve problems if any arose at work, and she could leave the job if she needed to. The therapist gave her hope that she could learn through therapy to get satisfaction from her job, and not feel so anxious, self-critical, and pained.

Another set of dysfunctional ideas that interfered with Patricia's willingness to consider getting a job related to her anger at her husband, who had told her when they got married that she could stay home and take care of their children and not have to work outside of the home. Patricia was angry that he had let her down and felt she should punish him. Her therapist helped her see that losing his job had been out of her husband's control. She acknowledged that he was doing everything he could to find another job and that he had taken a menial part-time job to try to keep the family afloat. Patricia was able, to some degree, to transfer her anger from him to their shared predicament.

Finally, Patricia revealed a strong coping strategy that she had employed since childhood, fantasizing about being rescued: "I want something or someone to take care of me." Her mother had been severely depressed when Patricia was young; her father worked long hours, drank from the moment he got home everyday, and was emotionally unavailable. As a child, she had wished to be rescued and had imagined someone—her mother, her father, a relative, or some unknown figure—swooping her up, showering her with attention and love, and taking care of her every need and desire. Now, 30 years later, she still hoped that somehow she would be saved: by her husband, by her therapist, or by someone yet unknown to her.

Patricia acknowledged that she felt let down that her therapist had not rescued her. She so wanted someone to arrange things so she could live a life of leisure, without distress. Her therapist empathized with the pain it caused Patricia that this scenario was unlikely to happen. In fact, she needed to mourn the loss of her fantasy, with support from her therapist, before she was willing to acknowledge that she needed to learn to take care of herself. Therapy notes helped remind her:

When I fantasize about being saved

There is no point in holding on to the rescue fantasy. It is destructive and in the long term causes me a lot of pain. If I work toward rescuing myself, I can have a better life. When I start to think that's not possible, remind myself that the depression is like a black mask over my face and makes me view my future in a depressed, unrealistic way.

Finally, Patricia was ready to start taking more steps toward getting better. By this time, the family's savings had been almost depleted and

Patricia saw no alternative to getting a job. Within 4 weeks of starting a job as a word processor, her depression plummeted. Although she did not particularly like the work, she could see how beneficial it was to her, and not only because it was providing much-needed income. Patricia recognized that having to go to her job took away her inner struggle about whether or not to do things. She no longer had a choice. She could not go back to bed, she had to organize herself in the morning, drop her son at school on the way to work, do the prescribed tasks, and make dinner for the family. Structuring her day, recognizing her accomplishments at work, experiencing positive interactions with her coworkers, receiving a reasonable response from her boss, and contributing to the well-being of her family were all important factors in lessening Patricia's depression. At first, she went back to her old habits on weekends, spending too much time in bed, not getting much done around the house. She herself decided to make changes. She had become convinced that she needed more structure.

Although her depressive symptoms had decreased almost to a normal level, Patricia was not yet ready to terminate. She needed more work on her dysfunctional beliefs about incompetence and unfairness and on relapse prevention.

WHEN PATIENTS DO NOT SEEM TO BE PROGRESSING

Finally, it is important to recognize that patients change at different rates. It may take time for new, adaptive ideas to sink in. Patients may need weeks—and in some cases, months—to contemplate what change means to them, to reveal their fears about change to the therapist, to address their fears, to see clearly the advantages of change, and to counter the disadvantages of change. And some patients simply are not ready to make needed changes when they present for treatment, especially if their emotional pain is relatively low. When patients make little or no movement after a period of time, they often do well to take a hiatus from therapy.

Before exploring the advantages and disadvantages of taking a break from treatment, however, therapists need to make sure that they are implementing therapy as effectively as possible and/or that they are not themselves having a negative reaction to the patient (as described in Chapter 6). Therapists need to evaluate and respond to ideas such as: "[The patient's] problems really are insoluble. She *should* be depressed, given her problems. She's resisting me. She isn't giving me a chance. I can't help her enough." They then should consider consultation to see if they can be more effective with the patient.

WHEN IT IS IMPORTANT NOT TO DO PROBLEM SOLVING

Although problem solving is an integral part of cognitive therapy, there are times when it is inappropriate: when patients are grieving a loss, when an emphasis on problem solving impacts negatively on the therapeutic relationship, and when patients bring up problems over which they have little or no control.

When patients have suffered a loss (which may be concrete or symbolic), therapists should offer support and validation. It is important that the therapist acknowledge the loss and support the grieving process. Talking about the meaning of the loss is often important. Therapists should intervene, however, when patients become unduly harsh with themselves or need immediate help coping more effectively.

It may be important to postpone problem solving when the therapist judges, based on data from the patient, that to do so will endanger the therapeutic alliance. When patients resist taking a problem-solving approach, the therapist needs to step back, conceptualize the problem, and first repair the alliance, as described in Chapters 4 and 5.

Finally, it is important to help patients recognize that they can not solve all problems. A patient with an alcoholic spouse, for example, may believe that he should be able to control his wife's drinking. A patient with an upset child may believe that she should be able to protect her child from feeling any distress. A patient from a dysfunctional family may believe that he should be able to make everyone get along with one another. Having examined the evidence and determining that patients do not have sufficient control, the therapist needs to help patients recognize that they may have to accept the existence of these problems, and work on their associated assumptions, for example, "If I can't fix this problem, it means [something bad about me]."

SUMMARY

A major thrust of cognitive therapy treatment is to help patients feel and function better in the coming week, which necessitates working toward solving problems and motivating patients to follow through with self-help assignments at every session. When patients have difficulty doing these essential therapy tasks, therapists need to specify the problem, then assess whether they themselves implemented standard strategies ineffectively and/or whether patients' dysfunctional beliefs interfered, necessitating a variation in the therapist's approach.

CHAPTER 10

Challenges in Identifying Cognitions

Most patients do not enter therapy with an understanding of the cognitive model: they are unaware that not only do their perceptions of situations influence how they react (emotionally, behaviorally, physiologically), but also that their thoughts are ideas (not necessarily truths), that their thoughts may be distorted, and that by evaluating and responding to their thinking they can feel better and behave more functionally. Often patients believe that difficult situations or other people *directly* affect their reactions. Or they may be mystified by their distress, unable to account for why it occurs. It is important for patients to understand the impact of their thinking on their reactions; otherwise, it will not make sense to them to engage in the process of eliciting (and responding to) their cognitions.

Even when patients do understand the cognitive model, they may struggle to identify their thoughts, images, assumptions, and core beliefs. When therapists ask them what was going through their mind (when they were distressed, behaving in a dysfunctional way, and/or experiencing distressing physical symptoms), patients may say that they do not know or that they were not thinking anything. They may change the subject, reply with an overintellectualized answer, or even refuse to speak. They may also exhibit these behaviors when the therapist is trying to ascertain the meaning of their thoughts in order to elicit underlying beliefs. As with any other problem in therapy, when patients have difficulty identifying their cognitions, therapists need to conceptualize why the problem has arisen so the therapist can plan an appropriate strategy.

Some difficulties in eliciting patients' dysfunctional cognitions are due to ineffective or inappropriate implementation of standard techniques, though sometimes therapists do need to vary standard approaches. This chapter describes how to elicit the automatic thoughts, images, assumptions, and beliefs of patients with challenging problems; the next three chapters describe how to modify these cognitions.

RECOGNIZING AUTOMATIC THOUGHTS

It is important for therapists to recognize that there is a range of situations that engender automatic thoughts, that a dearth of reported automatic thoughts may be related to patients' low symptomatology or to their avoidance, that automatic thoughts may be embedded in patients' discourse, and that patients may label their automatic thoughts as "feelings."

Recognizing the Range of Situations That Evoke Automatic Thoughts

Many "situations" can evoke automatic thoughts, as described in Chapter 2. Andrea's therapist, for example, was 10 minutes late for their session (situation 1). Andrea thought, "She doesn't really care about me," and felt hurt. She recognized her hurt feeling (situation 2), thought "How dare she make me feel bad!", and became angry. When she entered the therapist's office she expressed her anger. Before the therapist even spoke, Andrea recognized that she had overreacted (situation 3), and thought, "I shouldn't have said that. [My therapist] might not want to work with me any more."

Patients may have automatic thoughts about specific events, about their own thoughts (including those in verbal and imaginal form: daydreams, memories, fantasies), and about their reactions; (emotional, behavioral, and physiological responses). Patients may also have automatic thoughts about changes in their mind or body—for example, racing thoughts or physical pain. Or they may have thoughts about the stimulation of their senses: visual (such as visual hallucinations), auditory (such as auditory hallucinations), olfactory (such as smells that remind them of a traumatic experience), or kinesthetic (such as an unpleasant sensation from touch).

Recognizing When Patients Are Experiencing Few Negative Thoughts

Therapists may have difficulty eliciting automatic thoughts from patients whose symptoms are relatively mild. Patients who are in partial or full remission of an Axis I disorder, for example, generally have few current dysfunctional thoughts and therapy might focus at least partially on dysfunctional thoughts they predict they might have in the future (see J. Beck, 1995, for relapse-prevention techniques).

Recognizing Behavioral Avoidance

Some patients experience few automatic thoughts because they have a pervasive pattern of avoidance. Joel avoided putting himself in situations where he predicted he might be evaluated by others. He worked at home and stayed in as much as possible. When he had to go out, he would try to limit his exposure to other people; for example, he did errands when he thought stores would be least crowded. Initially, he only reported hopeless automatic thoughts about never being able to have a fulfilling life. (His therapist actually had little difficulty eliciting automatic thoughts when she discussed behavioral activation with him. Joel had many, many thoughts predicting negative outcomes.)

Recognizing Cognitive Avoidance

Patients who do not show significant *behavioral* avoidance, though, may still report few automatic thoughts if they routinely engage in *cognitive* avoidance, that is, pushing away thoughts that lead them to feel upset. Typically these patients try to distract themselves when they feel distressed so they won't focus on their thoughts and feel worse. They may engage in activities such as surfing the Internet, picking up a magazine, starting a conversation, walking around, getting something to eat, drinking alcohol or taking drugs (see Beck et al., 2004).

Recognizing Automatic Thoughts in Patients' Discourse

Sometimes patients express their thoughts in their description of an experience but they or their therapist do not realize it. In the transcript below, the therapist has to be alert for these thoughts, since the patient initially denied having had automatic thoughts.

THERAPIST: What were you thinking as you were talking to your mother on the phone?

PATIENT: Nothing, I was just so angry. You know, she *always* does this to me. She knows how upset I get when she talks about how I dropped out of school. I think she does it on purpose. She's always trying to needle me.

THERAPIST: (*summarizing*) So the situation was you were talking to your mother on the phone and you thought, "She always does this to me. She knows I get upset when she talks about school. Maybe she's doing it on purpose. She's needling me." And these thoughts led you to feel angry. Is that right?

Recognizing Automatic Thoughts Labeled as Feelings

Sometimes patients label their automatic thoughts as "feelings." When the patient uses the word "feelings," the therapist needs to conceptualize whether the patient has expressed an emotion or an idea.

THERAPIST: What did it mean to you that she always does this to you?

PATIENT: I don't know. I just feel so helpless, like I can never win with her.

THERAPIST: And when you have these thoughts, "I am helpless; I can't win with her," how do you feel emotionally?

PATIENT: Frustrated.

Relabeling the patient's ideas as thoughts and changing the patient's word "feel" to "feel emotionally" helps make the distinction clearer.

USING AND VARYING STANDARD STRATEGIES TO ELICIT AUTOMATIC THOUGHTS

Therapists employ a number of techniques to help patients identify their automatic thoughts, including using various forms of questioning, focusing on emotions and somatic sensations, using imagery, and using role play.

Questioning

The customary questions therapists use to elicit patients' automatic thoughts are:

> ■ "What was going through your mind?"
> ■ "What were you thinking?"

These questions, however, simply do not resonate with some patients, at least not initially. Therapists often need to be gently persistent in helping patients identify their automatic thoughts—being careful, of course, not to irritate patients or make them feel inadequate. They might ask:

> ■ "What were you imagining/ predicting/ remembering?"
> ■ "What did the situation mean to you?"
> ■ "What was the worst part of the situation?"

Therapists also might help patients to focus on their thoughts more clearly by first asking them to identify and focus somatically on their emotional reaction and then probing for their thoughts:

> ■ "How were you feeling emotionally?"
> ■ "Where did you feel the [emotion] in your body?"

Therapists can also provide a multiple-choice question, based on their conceptualization of the patient:

> ■ "Do you think you might have been thinking about _____ or _____?"

They might probe for patients' explanations for their reported emotion:

> ■ "You felt [sad] because you were thinking . . . ?"

or provide a thought *opposite* to the one they believe the patient actually had:

THERAPIST: Well, I bet you *weren't* thinking how wonderful things are?

PATIENT: No!

THERAPIST: What were you thinking?

PATIENT: That my life stinks! I hate my job!

Or the therapist might provide possibilities, using the thoughts they themselves might have:

> ■ "If I were in your situation, I might think _____. Does that ring a bell?"

Or thoughts others might have:

> ■ "You know, I hear from other people in this kind of situation that they sometimes think things like _____. Do you think you might have had thoughts like that?"

The following transcript illustrates the importance of being gently persistent and asking for thoughts in different ways. Note that it was not until the therapist realized that she did not have enough information about the distressing situation that she was able to supply the patient with a multiple-choice question, which finally enabled him to report his thoughts.

THERAPIST: (*summarizing*) So you were trying to e-mail your sister and you began to feel bad. What was going through your mind?

PATIENT: Nothing. Nothing. (*pause*) I just felt bad. Really bad.

THERAPIST: Bad, meaning . . . ?

PATIENT: Upset.

THERAPIST: (*probing for specific emotion*) Sad? Angry? Anxious? Confused?

PATIENT: I don't know, it was just a terrible feeling.

THERAPIST: (*probing for an image*) Did you have a picture in your mind?

PATIENT: No, just a blank.

THERAPIST: (*supplying an opposite thought*) You *weren't* thinking, "This is great. I'm so glad to be e-mailing my sister."

PATIENT: No.

THERAPIST: (*probing for a memory*) Could you have been remembering something?

PATIENT: I don't know.

THERAPIST: Well, this one is hard to figure out . . . (*realizing she needs more information*) I guess I should go back. Why were you e-mailing your sister?

PATIENT: I had to discuss something with her—about Mom—and I knew [automatic thought] she'd get really upset. That's why I was e-mailing her instead of calling.

THERAPIST: So, as you were sitting there, writing the e-mail, were you imagining how your sister would react?

PATIENT: I don't know. I was just feeling so bad.

THERAPIST: (*empathically*) Yeah, it must have been an upsetting e-mail to write. (*pause*) What's the worst part of the whole situation?

PATIENT: (*in a hopeless voice*) I don't know.

THERAPIST: (*offering multiple choice*) Something about your mom? About what you have to do? About having to deal with your sister?

PATIENT: (*looking defeated*) Everything. I'm so overwhelmed.

THERAPIST: (*in an empathic tone*) Could we talk about those things for a minute?

PATIENT: (*Nods.*)

THERAPIST: So there's your mom. Tell me about that part.

PATIENT: [automatic thoughts] I don't know what to do. She seems to be failing. I don't know if her doctor is treating her right.

THERAPIST: And your sister?

PATIENT: [automatic thoughts] She's so difficult. She wants to make every little decision about Mom, but she's not even here! She doesn't really know what's going on. She's always telling me I have to do this or I have to do that. And criticizing me. She has no idea how hard this whole thing is.

THERAPIST: And you? What's the effect of all this on you?

PATIENT: I'm just so overwhelmed. [automatic thoughts] I have to take care of my daughter. Meanwhile, if I want to keep my job, I have to work double shifts. Mom's medical bills are so expensive. She's almost run out of savings. I don't know what's going to happen!

THERAPIST: Anything else?

PATIENT: [automatic thoughts] My health hasn't been too good lately. I don't have time to take care of myself.

THERAPIST: (*reinforcing cognitive model, in empathic tone of voice*) Well, no wonder you were feeling so badly when you were trying to e-mail your sister. You were having all these upsetting thoughts about your mom, your sister, your daughter, yourself.

Focusing on Emotions and Somatic Sensations

When patients have difficulty identifying their thoughts, therapists can ask them to focus on their emotions and associated sensations. Doing so may increase their sensations and heighten their emotions, which may lead to easier access to their thoughts.

Stan was a 49-year-old man with obsessive–compulsive disorder. During their first session, when Stan's therapist asked him about his compulsions, he clutched his stomach and looked anxious.

THERAPIST: What just went through your mind?

STAN: I don't know.

THERAPIST: How are you feeling emotionally?

STAN: (*Thinks.*) Anxious.

THERAPIST: You put your hand on your stomach. Are you feeling uncomfortable?

STAN: (*Thinks.*) Yeah.

THERAPIST: What does your stomach feel like?

STAN: Like butterflies, only it hurts a little.

THERAPIST: Are you having any other symptoms?

STAN: Yeah, my chest feels tight.

THERAPIST: Can you focus on the anxiety and the feelings in your stomach and chest?

STAN: Yeah.

THERAPIST: When I asked you, "What do you do when you feel contaminated with germs," what were you thinking?

STAN: That if I tell you, you'll say I have to stop washing. I don't think I could stand doing that.

Some patients, whose automatic thoughts lead to a physiological reaction, are highly focused on changes in their body or mind and have little awareness of or deny that they are experiencing negative emotions or thoughts. It may be useful to teach these patients to identify their thoughts *after* they experience a somatic sensation, for example, "Oh, no, [the pain] is here again; it's probably going to get much worse," or "I can't stand [these symptoms]." Patients may then understand better how thoughts such as these may intensify their distress. Then therapists can ask patients to monitor situations in which they experience symptoms and together they can look for patterns. For example, Carl frequently reported abdominal distress shortly after waking up in the morning, when he first got to work, and at the end of the workday. By supplying him with hypothetical opposite thoughts, the patient was able to identify the anxiety-provoking thoughts he actually experienced.

Using Imagery

Another technique that is useful when patients are unable to identify their automatic thoughts involves imagery. Cynthia's therapist had already tried, without success, several different ways to elicit her thoughts about a situation that had happened earlier in the week.

THERAPIST: Can you imagine the scene again, as if it's happening right now? Can you try to see it in your mind? (*summarizing*) It was late Tuesday night and you were lying in bed?

CYNTHIA: Yeah.

THERAPIST: Can you describe it to me with some details? Where were you lying? What were you doing? How were you feeling?

CYNTHIA: I was still in my clothes, lying on my stomach. I was propped up on my elbows, I guess, because I was trying to read a magazine.

THERAPIST: Can you picture this as if it is happening right now? You're in your clothes. You're lying in bed, trying to read the magazine, propped up on your elbows. How are you feeling?

CYNTHIA: Incredibly down.

THERAPIST: Are you thinking about what you're reading?

CYNTHIA: No, I don't even *know* what I'm reading. I can't concentrate. In fact, I throw the magazine down.

THERAPIST: Can you see yourself throwing the magazine down?

CYNTHIA: Yeah.

THERAPIST: And you're thinking . . . ?

CYNTHIA: Oh, my god, I can't even focus on this stupid story.

THERAPIST: Which means . . . ?

CYNTHIA: There is something terribly wrong with me. (*pause*) I think I felt broken.

Using Role Play

Recreating an upsetting interpersonal situation in session can help patients gain better access to their thoughts. Carol had briefly described an argument she had had with her son, but despite the therapist's careful questioning, she was unable to figure out what she had been thinking.

THERAPIST: (*summarizing*) So your son was yelling at you. What was he saying?

CAROL: That he hates me. See, I told him he couldn't go to the mall with his friends. And then he started saying how I'm strangling him, that I never let him do things he wants.

THERAPIST: And what did you say back?

CAROL: I told him not to talk to me that way. But he kept arguing and arguing.

THERAPIST: I wonder if we could do a little role play, try to recreate the situation?

CAROL: Okay.

THERAPIST: Okay, how about if you play yourself and I'll play your son. As we're talking, try to figure out what you are thinking.

CAROL: Okay.

THERAPIST: How about if I start? Mom, I want to go to the mall with my friends.

CAROL: No, you can't.

THERAPIST: (*angrily*) Come on, Mom. Let me go!

CAROL: No, I told you that you couldn't. You haven't done your homework and it's a school night.

THERAPIST: I'll finish it when I get back.

CAROL: No, you can't go.

THERAPIST: Mom, you're strangling me! You never let me do anything I want! I hate you! I hate you!

CAROL: (*out of role play*) I think I turned away and started to cry.

THERAPIST: What was going through your mind?

CAROL: That Charlie is impossible! I can't stand the way he talks to me. He never listens. This is going on and on. I don't know if I have the strength to deal with him any more. And I know it's all my fault. I spoiled him when he was younger.

PROBLEMS IN IDENTIFYING AUTOMATIC THOUGHTS

A number of problems can arise when trying to help patients identify their automatic thoughts. They may supply intellectualized responses, they may be overly perfectionistic, or they may supply superficial thoughts. They may avoid identifying their thoughts because they fear that they will be overwhelmed with negative emotion, that their thoughts indicate something negative about them, or that their therapist will hurt them. (Note that these same problems can also arise when therapists attempt to identify images, assumptions, and core beliefs.)

When Patients Supply Intellectualized Responses

Sometimes patients overintellectualize and initially have difficulty identifying the actual thoughts that go through their minds. Asking for details about the distressing situation can often provide clues to what their automatic thoughts actually were. When Len has difficulty reporting his thoughts, the therapist offers a tentative hypothesis, based on further information the patient supplied:

THERAPIST: So you were feeling the most uncomfortable before dinner started?

LEN: Yeah.

THERAPIST: What was going through your mind?

LEN: Well, it was a question of intimacy, a fear of intimacy.

THERAPIST: And what did you predict would happen?

LEN: Nothing. It's just this idea of intimacy; it's uncomfortable for me.

THERAPIST: Who were you feeling the most uncomfortable around?

LEN: (*Thinks.*) Not my kids. My sister-in-law, I guess.

THERAPIST: And you were thinking, "She'll probably . . . ?"

LEN: . . . Try to talk to me.

THERAPIST: About . . . ?

LEN: Maybe just small talk. But she'll ask me what I'm doing.

THERAPIST: And that could be bad?

LEN: Well, I can't impress her any more with my (*in an ironic voice*) dazzling achievements.

THERAPIST: So, she might think or say . . . ?

LEN: I don't know. It actually didn't happen. She was busy helping out in the kitchen. I never did really talk to her.

THERAPIST: But, if you *had* talked to her, it wouldn't have made you feel good?

LEN: No.

THERAPIST: Okay, let me know if I got this about right. The situation was that the family had gathered in the living room before dinner. And you were thinking about talking to your sister-in-law and you had some kind of thought like "She's going to ask me about what I've been doing and that will make me feel bad." Is that right?

LEN: Yeah.

When Patients Are Overly Perfectionistic

Some patients are concerned that if the therapist does not have a full and completely accurate understanding of their automatic thoughts, he or she will not be able to help them. So they are overly concerned with giving the therapist the "right answer" about their automatic thoughts, reflecting too much before answering. They may try to report every thought, overwhelming themselves and their therapist. Or they may continually correct their therapist when he or she is summarizing their thoughts. Unless they have overly rigid assumptions about the need to be perfectly understood, they often just need psychoeducation.

THERAPIST: What would happen if you just took a guess about your thoughts [or "if you didn't report every thought" or "if I didn't summarize your thoughts exactly right"]?

PATIENT: (*pause*) I'm not sure.

THERAPIST: Are you worried that I might not understand well enough?

PATIENT: Yes, yes, I think so.

THERAPIST: So let me reassure you. I just need to get a *general* idea of what your problems are and what your thoughts are. I don't need to know everything and I don't necessarily need to know the details. I just have to get the general impression. (*pause*) How much do you believe me, when I tell you it's okay if you don't give me perfect answers [or "if I don't get the details right"]?

PATIENT: I don't know. I guess I thought you *wouldn't* be able to help me.

THERAPIST: You know, that's not been my experience. How about just trying to give me an overall picture and at the end of session we'll see how it went?

When Patients Supply Superficial Automatic Thoughts

Some patients report only "coping" thoughts—rationalizations or false reassurances—that they say to make themselves feel better *after* their initial upsetting thoughts. Ron often reported such thoughts. Ron's therapist asked him what went through his mind when his friend didn't ask him to go to a basketball game. Ron reported, "I didn't really want to go anyway." Upon further questioning, his therapist discovered that Ron's initial automatic thought actually had been "He must not like me any more." Another time Ron related feeling very anxious when his wife was late returning from work. He identified his thoughts as "She'll be all right. She'll be all right." This "coping" statement (which was, at best, only minimally helpful) came to mind after an original thought and image about his wife's being in an accident.

Other patients offer superficial automatic thoughts when there are far more important cognitions below the surface. In the following transcript, the therapist again has to probe to elicit the patient's more distressing thoughts:

THERAPIST: So are you going to go back to work today?

PATIENT: (*slowly*) No . . . I don't think so.

THERAPIST: Because . . . ?

PATIENT: I really don't want to go [superficial thought].

THERAPIST: What's the worst thing that could happen if you go?

PATIENT: Nothing.

THERAPIST: How do you feel when you think about going?

PATIENT: Not great. It's . . . it's frustrating. You know, I'm leaving the job. They really don't appreciate me there.

THERAPIST: Are you going to go tomorrow?

PATIENT: Yeah, I'll go tomorrow.

THERAPIST: But tomorrow will be frustrating, too, won't it?

PATIENT: Yeah. But I have some home things I have to get done.

THERAPIST: So is there something that bothers you about going *today* and not getting those home things done *today*?

PATIENT: (*Sighs.*)

THERAPIST: (*hypothesizing, based on a previously identified pattern*) I wonder if somewhere in the back of your mind is the idea that you ought to be careful today, take care of yourself. Even though you know intellectually that you're okay, that nothing will happen, maybe you think you should be on the safe side and not exert yourself?

PATIENT: I don't know. (*Thinks.*) I guess I do think I'd be better off if I went home and took a nap.

THERAPIST: Because if you're not careful and don't take a nap but go to work instead . . . ?

PATIENT: It might not be good for me.

THERAPIST: And the worst thing that might happen?

PATIENT: I don't know. (*pause*) My supervisor might give me a hard time again.

THERAPIST: And if he did, then what could happen?

PATIENT: I just don't want to get upset.

THERAPIST: Because if you got too upset . . . ?

PATIENT: I guess I could go way downhill.

Now the patient's key automatic thought is clear: "[If I go to work today, my supervisor might give me a hard time and] I'll get too upset and go way downhill."

When Patients Display a Pattern of Cognitive (and Emotional) Avoidance

Some patients avoid reporting—and sometimes even recognizing—automatic thoughts that are distressing because of their fear of experiencing negative emotion. They may hold a belief such as "If I think about this, I'll feel worse (I'll be overwhelmed, lose control of my emotions, fall apart, go crazy)." In addition, patients sometimes have images that accompany these thoughts. They may envision themselves overcome with emotion. Often therapists need to determine whether the patient has a dysfunctional assumption such as this and evaluate it before the patient is willing to identify distressing cognitions. Lorraine's former boyfriend had purposely ignored her at a bar. This happened several days before her next therapy session and she had ruminated about the incident and felt quite pained ever since. When her therapist asked her about it, Lorraine had an image of herself revealing the information, then crying and crying, without being able to stop.

THERAPIST: Okay, should we talk about what happened to you when you saw Travis?

LORRAINE: (*Looks down.*) I don't think I should talk about it now.

THERAPIST: Well, that's okay. But can you tell me what you think could happen if you did tell me about it?

LORRAINE: I don't know. I'd probably get too upset.

THERAPIST: Do you have a picture in your mind of what would happen if you got too upset?

LORRAINE: (*Thinks.*) Yeah, I'd just cry and cry and cry.

THERAPIST: And then what would happen?

LORRAINE: I don't know.

THERAPIST: What's your worst fear?

LORRAINE: That I'd never stop crying, I guess. Have a total nervous break-down.

Her therapist next asked her to recall whether something similar had ever previously happened to her in therapy. Lorraine replied that it had not. Then he asked her to relate times when she had focused on her thoughts and become too upset. Lorraine briefly described two incidents in recent months when she was alone in her apartment at night and cried on and off for over an hour. Her therapist helped her see that even at those times she had eventually stopped crying and had not experienced "a nervous breakdown." They also discussed how her experience would likely be different here in their session, because Lorraine was not alone, and she and the therapist would focus on alleviating her pain. Her therapist then had Lorraine recall times in therapy when talking about an upsetting incident had helped her feel better, not worse. At the end of this discussion, Lorraine was willing to talk about the incident with her ex-boyfriend. Toward the end of the session, the therapist helped Lorraine conclude that discussing the problem with him had indeed led to an improvement in her mood.

A graded exposure approach is indicated for some patients who are reluctant to identify their automatic thoughts. Therapists might ask these patients to reveal just one part of an incident to see what does happen to them. Or they might ask patients to focus on their negative thoughts for just a few seconds or minutes, then gradually build up the amount of time they can tolerate reflecting on their negative thoughts. Additional techniques for addressing a fear of experiencing negative emotion are presented in Chapter 12.

When Patients Put a Special Meaning to Their Thoughts

Patients may be reluctant to report their thoughts because of the meaning they attach to them. Drew did not want to admit his fears of traveling beyond his comfort zone because he did not want to see himself as weak. Tyler was worried that his obsessive thoughts meant that he was crazy. Jeremy disparaged himself for having negative thoughts about his prospects in his sales job: "Only losers think like this." When therapists sense such reluctance, it is important to ask patients:

■ "Do you think there's something bad about thinking in this way?"

Then therapists can help them reframe the negative connotation they have attached to their thoughts.

When Patients Fear Their Therapists' Response

A failure to identify cognitions is sometimes related to problems in the therapeutic relationship (see Chapters 4 and 5). Patients may avoid disclosing automatic thoughts because they feel too vulnerable to their therapist:

"If I tell my therapist what I was thinking, [he/she] will . . . ."
- "Think I'm crazy/pitiful/repugnant/beyond help."
- "Criticize me, put me down, reject me."
- "Report me to the police/send me to the hospital/refuse to see me again."
- "Control me/use it against me in some way."

When therapists suspect a problem in the alliance, they can ask the patient directly about their hypothesis:

■ "If you tell me what you are thinking, could something bad happen?"
■ "Do you think I might judge you negatively in some way?"

Some patients are reluctant to express their concerns, however, and the therapist may need to negotiate with them.

Case Example

In his first therapy session, Don, a 52-year-old man with chronic depression, did not want to identify his automatic thoughts for fear the therapist would think he was stupid or weak. Instead of answering her question about his automatic thoughts during an upsetting incident at work, he put his therapist down. She had to help him feel more in control before he was willing to collaborate on identifying his thinking.

DON: You know, all this focus on my thoughts isn't very helpful. It's so superficial.

THERAPIST: Hmmm. (*pause*) Do you have a sense of what would help you more?

DON: (*not really answering the question*) You see, my problems are really very deep-seated. I have felt depressed my entire life. And no one has been able to help me, I mean, not for long. I'm sure it has to do with how neglectful my parents were. I didn't get what I needed. And that's still affecting me today. So talking about this stuff, it's, it's . . . trivial.

THERAPIST: I can see why it would seem that way. (*empathizing*) And I would imagine it must be irritating to you.

DON: Well, yes. I had thought you would work at a deeper level.

THERAPIST: You're absolutely right. We *do* have to work at a deeper level. It's just a question of timing. Most people don't make much progress if we *start* at a deep level. It's like trying to start off running a marathon when you haven't exercised for a year. Usually it's better to start off just walking a few blocks and build muscle without injuring yourself.

DON: I still think talking about what I was thinking at work just won't be very productive.

THERAPIST: Well, you may be right about that . . . or you may be wrong. But I would certainly be willing to split our time in therapy—spending some time on upsetting situations like work and spending some time on deeper issues, like what happened with your parents. (*pause*) What do you think?

DON: (*Thinks, in a reluctant voice.*) I suppose so.

THERAPIST: Should we start with your childhood experiences then?

The therapist then split the time between his childhood experiences and teaching him the cognitive model, using the incident at work as an example.

POSTPONING THE IDENTIFICATION OF AUTOMATIC THOUGHTS

Sometimes it is important *not* to persist in trying to help patients identify their automatic thoughts when doing so evokes negative thoughts about themselves, about the therapist, or about the process of therapy. At these times, therapists should downplay the importance of eliciting the thoughts in the particular situation:

> ■ "Sometimes these thoughts are hard to figure out. We may come back to this later." ["Meanwhile, can you tell me more about the problem?" or "Maybe we should talk about the problem you're having with _____ instead. What do you think?"]

If, however, therapists observe a *pattern* of difficulty in identifying cognitions, they should investigate whether there is still a practical problem or whether the patient has interfering beliefs, as described later in this chapter.

IDENTIFYING IMAGES

As described elsewhere (Beck, Emery, & Greenberg, 1985; J. Beck, 1995), most patients do not spontaneously report negative visual images. Since these images are frequently quite distressing, patients tend to push them out of their awareness very quickly. To compound the problem, many therapists fail even to *ask* patients about images, much less probe for them. It is important to identify patients' images, since they may experience insufficient relief if they are not addressed.

Images may be predictions, memories, or metaphorical representations.

Predictions

Patients' thoughts are often accompanied by images, as illustrated in the following examples. Danielle, a high school student, saw a group of girls from her school across the street. They seemed to be laughing and Danielle thought, "I'll bet they're talking about me." She was too far away to see them clearly or to hear them at all, but she had an image of their laughing meanly, with scornful expressions on their faces, agreeing with one another that Danielle was a "loser." Randy was quite nervous at work. When a coworker reminded him that his yearly evaluation was coming up, Randy thought, "I'm going to get a terrible evaluation." He had an image of his boss calling him into his office, criticizing him for not working hard enough, and firing him on the spot. When Brian's wife called him to say that his mother had to go back into the hospital, Brian thought, "What if she gets even sicker?" He imagined his mother expiring on her hospital bed. When Al became quite upset, he thought, "I can't stand feeling like this." He had an image of running down the street, screaming, and feeling totally out of control. Then he saw himself being forced into an ambulance by men in white coats.

Therapists can directly ask for images when they hear a prediction:

> ■ "When you have the thought,['I'll end up on the street'], do you have a picture in your mind of what that looks like?"

Or they can ask indirectly. Marjorie reported her thought "I'll never get better." Her therapist suggested,

> ■ "Let's say it's a few years from now and you don't feel better, where do you see yourself? What are you doing?"

Therapists can also assume that the patient has had an image and ask for visual details:

> ■ "So you had the thought 'When I get up in front of the room and try to talk, I won't be able to.' What did the room look like? Who was there? How were you feeling? How did you look? What was the audience thinking?"

Memories

Painful memories are often encapsulated in specific images. When Jenny felt confused, she sometimes had a spontaneous image of sitting in her first-grade class, feeling overwhelmed and humiliated because she was unable to understand a worksheet the teacher wanted her to complete.

In session, Teresa's therapist asked for evidence that she would not be able to survive if her husband died. She reported a visual memory from several years before when she had moved out of her parents' house to live alone for the first time. It was her first night in her new apartment and she was feeling sad, lonely, and extremely overwhelmed.

Metaphorical Representations

Sometimes patients have spontaneous images that are metaphorical in nature. Mitchell related, "When I think about trying to make changes in my life, I don't know, it's like I'm running into a wall." Indeed he saw himself painfully bouncing off a tall, forbidding brick wall. Carla told her therapist about the overwhelming pain she had experienced during the week and said, "I felt like I was drowning." When questioned, her therapist ascertained that Carla had had an image of sinking beneath the surface of a deep lake.

ELICITING ASSUMPTIONS

As described in Chapter 2, assumptions may be situation-specific ("If I try to get the kids to do that [take more responsibility around the house], it just won't work; they won't listen to me"). Or assumptions may be at a deeper, more general level ("If I try to influence others, I'll fail"). Assumptions, such as these two, may be predictive. Or assumptions may be more directly thematically tied to the core belief ("If I can't get people to listen to me, it shows I'm weak").

As described in earlier chapters, patients with challenging problems often have dysfunctional assumptions about making changes in general and changes in therapy, about the process of therapy, and about the therapist—for example:

- "If I try to make changes, I'll fail."
- "If I get better, my life will get worse."
- "If I discuss upsetting things, I'll get overwhelmed."
- "If I go along with my therapist, it will show I'm weak."

USING AND VARYING STANDARD STRATEGIES TO ELICIT ASSUMPTIONS

Most assumptions are fairly easy to identify: patients express them outright (e.g., "If I don't hound my partner, he'll never do anything"). Or the therapist can use one of the following techniques.

Providing Part of the Assumption

THERAPIST: (*summarizing*) So you feel bad when you think about not being able to help out at the shelter?

PATIENT: Yeah.

THERAPIST: Because "If I can't help out at the shelter . . . ." What? What does that mean? Or what could happen?

PATIENT: I've let them down.

The therapist may decide to go deeper and continue to ask for the meaning of the patients' assumptions ("And if you do let them down, that means . . . ?") until patients reveal their core beliefs.

Other strategies are presented below.

Providing a Sentence Stem

Once a therapist has identified a pattern of dysfunctional behavior, it is particularly helpful to ask the patient to complete assumptions that include the behavior:

- "If I [do my coping strategy], then _____ [what good thing happens or what good thing does it mean?]."
- "If I don't [do my coping strategy] then _____ [what bad thing happens or what bad thing does it mean?]."

For example, Patricia's therapist helped her identify both a small subset assumption (a prediction) and then the more general assumption tied to her core belief:

THERAPIST: Patricia, how would you answer this: If I have to do mundane chores like laundry and dishes and cleaning the bathroom, then what bad thing will happen?

PATRICIA: I'll be dragged down, no energy, it will feel endless.

THERAPIST: And what does it *mean* to you to have to do these mundane chores?

PATRICIA: I just feel small, trapped.

THERAPIST: (*gathering data to see if the assumption is just situation-specific or whether there is a deeper level assumption*) Do you feel that way about doing everything around the house?

PATRICIA: Most things. (*Thinks.*) Except baking, cooking—I like those things.

THERAPIST: So, it's doing things you feel obligated to do and don't like that are a problem?

PATRICIA: Yeah.

THERAPIST: And things out of the house? Is it similar?

PATRICIA: Yeah. I've always been like that.

THERAPIST: So, if I do things I don't want to do, it means I'm small, trapped. Is that right?

PATRICIA: Yeah, I think so.

Translating Attitudes and Rules into the Assumption Form

As described in Chapter 2, it is easier to conceptualize and test intermediate-level beliefs when they are in the form of an assumption, as opposed to attitudes and rules. In addition, assumptions often help make explicit the link between coping strategies and core beliefs. Liz's attitude was "It's terrible to make other people upset," and her rule was "I should never make other people upset." Her therapist asked her for the meaning of making others upset and Liz replied, "If I make other people upset, they might hurt me."

ELICITING CORE BELIEFS

Core beliefs may be elicited in various ways, as described below. It is important to recognize that the identification of core beliefs may be quite distressing to patients. Therapists may gingerly elicit these beliefs early in therapy to help them conceptualize patients but they must take care that patients do not feel too threatened or vulnerable by their doing so.

USING AND VARYING STANDARD STRATEGIES TO ELICIT CORE BELIEFS

Therapists can use a variety of techniques to identify patients' core beliefs. They can investigate the meaning of patients' thoughts, examine their assumptions, recognize when beliefs are expressed as automatic thoughts, or offer a list of core beliefs (see Chapter 2).

Asking for the Meaning of Patients' Thoughts

Therapists can examine themes embedded in patients' automatic thoughts across situations and across time and ask them for the *meaning* of their thoughts.

> ■ "If this automatic thought is true . . . ."
>   "What does that mean?"
>   "What is the worst part about the situation?"
>   "What's so bad about that?"
>   "What does that mean about you?"
>   "What does that mean about others or the world?"

If patients have difficulty with these questions, therapists can tentatively offer an educated guess, based on patterns they have observed in the patient's thinking.

THERAPIST: If it's true that your brother blames you for not helping care for your parents, what does that mean?

PATIENT: (*pause*) I'm not sure.

THERAPIST: What would be the worst part about it?

PATIENT: (*pause*) I don't know.

THERAPIST: Is it possible that you think he's right? That you do deserve blame?

PATIENT: Yeah, yeah.

THERAPIST: And if you do deserve blame . . . ?

PATIENT: (*Looks down.*)

THERAPIST: Does it mean that you're bad?

PATIENT: (*Whispers.*) Yes.

Examining Assumptions

Sometimes patients exhibit maladaptive assumptions that are situation-specific and not deeply rooted in their core beliefs. These assumptions are often readily modifiable. At other times patients' maladaptive assumptions are reflections of a more general core belief, which makes the problematic assumptions more difficult to change. Contrast two patients, both of whom hold the assumption "If I set limits with my friend, he won't like me anymore."

THERAPIST: And Robert, if it's true that your friend won't like you any more, what would that mean?

ROBERT: He won't want to be around me. I'll lose him as a friend.

THERAPIST: And if you lose him as a friend, what would that mean?

ROBERT: I wouldn't have him to hang out with any more. He's really a lot of fun to be with. I'd miss that.

THERAPIST: And what would that mean about you, if you lost him as a friend, didn't have him to hang out with and have fun with?

ROBERT: I guess I'd have to hang out with my other friends more.

THERAPIST: Would it say anything bad about *you*, if you lost him as a friend.

ROBERT: (*without much emotion*) No, I don't think so.

Robert did not have a core belief connected with his assumption that his friend wouldn't like him any more. Marcy, however, did.

THERAPIST: Marcy, if it's true that your friend won't like you any more, what would that mean?

MARCY: I'll lose him.

THERAPIST: And if you lose him as a friend, what would that mean?

MARCY: (*in a small voice*) I'll never find anyone else.

THERAPIST: What would that mean about you?

MARCY: I'm . . . unlovable.

THERAPIST: Is this an idea that you have a lot—or only connected to Bruce?

MARCY: I do feel that way a lot.

THERAPIST: For example . . . ?

MARCY: When I'm around my family, (*thinking*) when I'm at work, at church, at [my social group].

THERAPIST: When *don't* you feel unlovable?

MARCY: I don't know. Hardly ever. (*thinking*) Maybe when I'm around my niece.

Unlike Robert, Marcy had a core belief of unlovability that became acti-vated when she thought about being more assertive with her friend—and in countless instances across situations and across time.

Recognizing When Core Beliefs Are Expressed as Automatic Thoughts

Some patients easily identify their core beliefs early in treatment, espe-cially many depressed patients, who actually express their core beliefs as automatic thoughts ("I'm a failure. I'm no good. I feel so worthless"). Therapists can confirm whether these thoughts are core beliefs by deter-mining whether they are generalized ideas, not just situation-specific, as illustrated in the example above.

Specifying Ambiguous Core Beliefs

Some patients express general core beliefs about the self that are not easily categorized without further questioning: "There's something wrong with me," "I'm not good enough," "I'm defective." In order to conceptualize them better, therapists can question patients to determine whether their core belief is in the helpless, unlovable, or worthless cate-gory.

THERAPIST: And if people don't come up to you at the party, what would that mean?

PATIENT: They're ignoring me. They don't want to talk to me.

THERAPIST: And if it's true that they don't want to talk to you, what would that mean about you?

PATIENT: That there's something wrong with me.

THERAPIST: And if there *is* something wrong with you, what would be the worst part? That you're not as *good* as other people [belief of inferior-ity in the helpless category], that you'll never get the *love and intimacy* you want from other people [belief in the unlovability category], or that you're *bad or worthless*?

PATIENT: That I'm not as good as them. They're interesting, they have great jobs, most of them are married, some of them even have kids.

THERAPIST: And you?

PATIENT: I don't have any of those things.

THERAPIST: So what does that say about you?

PATIENT: I'm inferior.

PROBLEMS IN IDENTIFYING CORE BELIEFS

When the strategies described above are ineffective, it may be particularly difficult to identify patients' core beliefs, especially if they fear experiencing negative emotion or expect that their therapist could harm them. When asked for the meaning of their thoughts, these patients may continue to focus on more superficial automatic thoughts, or may seem perplexed and say, "I don't know." They may have hypotheses about their core beliefs, but feel too vulnerable and distressed to talk about them and thus avoid further discussion. When this happens, therapist should tread lightly, using a gradual, gentle exploratory approach.

SUMMARY

Patients may experience difficulty in identifying their automatic thoughts, images, assumptions, and core beliefs for a number of reasons. As with other difficulties, therapists should assess whether the problem seemed to arise because they were not able to use standard techniques effectively and/or whether they should have used alternative strategies, given patients' dysfunctional beliefs regarding thinking about or expressing their negative cognitions.

CHAPTER 11

Challenges in Modifying Thoughts and Images

An important part of cognitive therapy is changing patients' cognitions to bring about emotional, behavioral, and physiological change. Cognitive therapists often start working at the automatic thought level because this superficial level of cognition is more amenable to change than are underlying assumptions and core beliefs. Modification of underlying beliefs is undertaken as quickly as possible because once patients experience a fundamental change in their distorted views of themselves, their worlds, and others, they tend to have fewer distorted thoughts, feel better emotionally, and behave more functionally. Trying to help some patients with challenging problems evaluate their beliefs at the beginning of treatment, though, is often unsuccessful.

Robin, for example, has a core belief that she is bad and defective and that others are likely to be critical of her and rejecting. If her therapist could help her change these beliefs at the first session—if Robin could immediately start to believe that she was worthwhile, normal, okay, and that others were likely to be benign and accepting—she would have many fewer negative thoughts about herself and many fewer fears of how other people would see and treat her. She would then be likely to engage in more functional behavior and her mood would improve. Robin's core beliefs, however, are so tenacious that it does not make sense to her to question them. If her therapist tries too soon to help her evaluate this negative view of herself, Robin may become quite confused and anxious or she may believe that her therapist doesn't understand her, has nefarious purposes, or is naive and incompetent.

Some automatic thoughts and images of patients with challenging problems are relatively easy to modify; some, especially those more closely linked with patients' underlying beliefs, are more difficult. The first part of this chapter contains standard strategies with variations to help patients modify their automatic thoughts *in* session. Then typical beliefs that lead patients to resist modifying their thoughts are presented. The second part of the chapter discusses modifying automatic thoughts *between* sessions.

USING AND VARYING STANDARD STRATEGIES TO MODIFY AUTOMATIC THOUGHTS

Patients with challenging problems, unless they are behaviorally or cognitively avoidant, may have dozens or hundreds of automatic thoughts in the course of a week. Therapists need a good working conceptualization (see Chapter 2) to help them collaboratively decide with patients which problem(s) to focus on during a given session—and, in the context of discussing a problem, which relatively few automatic thoughts to evaluate and try to modify during that session.

Before Initiating the Evaluation Process

Prior to beginning the process of helping patients evaluate their thinking, therapists need to ensure that they are addressing *key* automatic thoughts, and that patients still believe their automatic thoughts to a significant degree. Therapists also need to recognize that significant cognitive change is often not brought about when patients' associated affect is low.

Selecting Key Automatic Thoughts

In selecting automatic thoughts (or images) to evaluate with the patient, therapists need to establish which of the dozens or hundreds of automatic thoughts that patients had during the week are most important to modify. Alternatively, therapists and patients may focus on key automatic thoughts they predict the patient is likely to experience in the coming week. It is desirable to select thoughts that:

- Are associated with the problem they are addressing in session.
- Are quite typical of the patient.
- Are significantly distorted or dysfunctional.
- Are reflective of an important underlying belief.
- Are associated with significant negative affect (J. Beck, 1995).

Ascertaining the Degree of Belief in the Automatic Thought

Before evaluating an automatic thought, therapists should ask questions such as the following:

■ "How much do you believe this [automatic thought] right now?"
■ "How much do you believe it intellectually? How much emotionally?"

If patients' degree of belief is relatively low at both an intellectual and an emotional level, therapists may simply ask patients:

■ "Were you able to answer back that thought?"
■ "How do you see it *now*?"

If patients have already changed their thinking, further cognitive restructuring may not be required. For example, Marlene had been quite upset when she realized that she would have to tell her son that she could not baby-sit for his children the following week because she had a doctor's appointment. Her key automatic thoughts during the previous week had been "I should do this for him. He's counting on me. I'm really letting him down." Fortunately, her therapist checked with her, found out that she no longer believed these thoughts very much, and recognized that she did not need his help responding to them.

THERAPIST: How much do you believe *right now* that you should do this for him instead of keeping your doctor's appointment and that you're letting him down?

MARLENE: Not that much, I guess.

THERAPIST: How do you see it now?

MARLENE: That in the scheme of things, it isn't so bad. I do a lot of baby-sitting for him already. And it's not like I'm canceling so I can go to the movies or something.

THERAPIST: That's good. I'm glad you can see it that way.

Marlene's therapist then conceptualized that their time would be better spent on automatic thoughts or problems that were more distressing to the patient.

Ensuring an Appropriate Degree of Negative Affect

Patients' affect may be low if:

- They have already changed their thinking (as was the case with Marlene, above).
- They are cognitively avoidant.
- Their distress is evoked only when they are in the upsetting situation itself.

Therapists who have patients in the last two groups need to heighten patients' affect, often by asking them to imagine the situation as if it is happening right now.

On the other hand, occasionally patients' affect is *too* high for them to evaluate their thinking. Usually their core beliefs have become strongly activated in the therapy session itself. Therapists may need to change the subject or encourage the patient to use relaxation, slow-breathing, or distraction techniques, until the patient is feeling less distressed and more in control, before returning to the original automatic thought.

Using Standard Questioning

The primary technique that therapists use to help patients modify their thinking is Socratic questioning. Therapists often use some of the following basic questions—or variations of them—to help patients evaluate their thinking:

- ■ "What's the evidence that this thought is true? What's the evidence on the other side that this thought might not be true, or not completely true?"
- ■ "What is an alternative explanation or a different way of looking at this situation?"
- ■ "What cognitive distortion might I be making?"
- ■ "What's the worst that could happen in this situation (and, if appropriate, how could I *cope* if it did happen)? What's the best that could happen? What's the most realistic outcome?"
- ■ "What is the effect of believing this automatic thought? What could happen if I changed my thinking?"
- ■ "What would I tell [a specific friend or family member] if he/she were in this situation and had this thought?"
- ■ "What should I do now?"

These questions are described in *Cognitive Therapy: Basics and Beyond*, (J. Beck, 1995) and can be found at the bottom of the Dysfunctional Thought Record (J. Beck, 2005). Note that not all questions are applicable to a given automatic thought. Christy, for example, thought, "I don't want to get up and start the day." That thought was patently true, so her therapist did not ask her the first three questions above.

Using Other Types of Questions and Techniques

Sometimes therapists need to use a number of techniques to help the patient gain a more functional perspective. Lucy was highly anxious about going to a singles event at her church. She had a host of automatic thoughts: "What if I don't know anyone? What if I don't know what to say? What if I blush and stutter? What if I sound foolish?" Her therapist used standard Socratic questioning to help her evaluate and respond to these thoughts. She ascertained that Lucy's anxiety seemed to be much more apparent to her than to other people and that Lucy did know appropriate things to say; she just felt inhibited. Following this discussion, Lucy felt less anxious. But her next automatic thought was "If I talk about myself, they'll think I'm conceited." Her therapist could have helped Lucy evaluate and respond to that thought by using standard questions:

- ■ "How do you know that they'd find you conceited? Have you had lots of past experiences where you know for sure that people found you conceited? Or have you actually been pretty quiet?"
- ■ "Is it possible that people would find you interesting and pleasant, but not conceited?"
- ■ "Could you be making a fortune-telling error?"
- ■ "What's the worst that could happen if people did find you conceited? What could you do if that happened? What's the best that could happen in this situation? What's the most realistic outcome of this situation?"
- ■ "What is the effect of believing that people will find you conceited? What could happen if you changed your thinking?"
- ■ "If your friend Daphne were in this situation and had this thought, what would you tell her?"
- ■ "What do you think you should do?"

There are a number of other ways that Lucy's therapist could address this automatic thought. For example, she might question Lucy in a *persuasive* way.

THERAPIST: So it sounds as if everyone there is single and is purposely going to meet other people?

LUCY: Yeah.

THERAPIST: So they're not going with the purpose of being mean to other people or putting them down or making them feel uncomfortable?

LUCY: (*Thinks.*) No, I guess not.

THERAPIST: Are there a lot of people like that at your church, anyway?

LUCY: Oh, no, it's a pretty accepting place.

THERAPIST: Is it possible there will be other shy people there?

LUCY: I guess so.

THERAPIST: If you were to go up to someone and start making conversation, do you think most people there would be annoyed or *glad* that someone is taking an interest in them?

LUCY: Maybe it would be all right.

The therapist could offer an *alternative perspective*:

THERAPIST: So you predict that people will consider you conceited if you talk about yourself. (*pause*) I wonder, Lucy, if the *opposite* might happen? You meet a guy there, you ask him some questions to show you're interested in him as a person. And if he's not good at asking you the same kind of questions back, you smooth the conversation by volunteering information about yourself: how long you've belonged to the church, what you like about the church, where you work . . . things like that. (*pause*) Maybe rather than seeing you as *conceited*, he'd be *grateful* that you're carrying the ball conversationally, especially if *he's* a little shy. (*pause*) What do you think?

She could also address the thought in a more *extreme* fashion to point out its distortion:

THERAPIST: You know, you're right in that you don't want to *overpower* him or *dominate* the whole conversation with how great you are—but honestly, Lucy, do you see that happening? I think we'd have to do a whole personality transplant for you to sound narcissistic or too self-important. (*pause*) Do you think I'm right?

Lucy's therapist could use *self-disclosure*:

THERAPIST: You know, when I'm talking to people socially, I feel uncomfortable if I have to do all the talking. Even if they seem interested and ask me lots of questions, it just feels unbalanced to me if they don't really volunteer anything or don't say much when I ask questions. I *like* it when they talk about themselves—unless, of course, they totally *monopolize* the whole conversation. (*pause*) What do you think of that?

Lucy's therapist might draw a *diagram* to help her understand this concept.

Doesn't talk about self at all	(	midrange	)	Dominates the conversation completely

THERAPIST: You see, I think most people aren't very comfortable when the other person is at either extreme of the continuum. What you might want to aim for is a range in the middle.

The therapist might also address the thought in an *experiential* way. She could ask Lucy to role-play a man she might meet at church and notice the man's reaction while the therapist took Lucy's role. In the first role play, the therapist, as Lucy, was very quiet, did not volunteer information, and just asked a few questions in a quiet voice, not making eye contact. In the second role play, the therapist played Lucy in a more outgoing fashion. After the role plays, they discussed how much more comfortable the second role play had been.

The therapist could do *imagery* work, described later in this chapter, with Lucy, identifying the distressing fantasy in her mind of what could happen at the church and replacing it with a more realistic image.

Lucy's therapist might also be forthrightly positive and *supportive*:

THERAPIST: You know, Lucy, I think people at church would be *lucky* if you were willing to talk to them. You're such a nice person!

Finally, Lucy and her therapist might set up a *behavioral experiment* for homework, one that her therapist predicts would be highly likely to be successful. Before she walked into the church social, Lucy would read her therapy notes (which contained conclusions she had drawn in the session and behavioral instructions about what to do). She would then try to talk to two people to test her belief that she would sound conceited. After the social, she would assess the degree to which her automatic thoughts had been accurate, using guidelines she and the therapist had developed in session (using people's tone of voice, facial expressions, and body language to judge whether they had had a positive or a neutral reaction to her—or whether they had had an overtly negative reaction). Just in case the behavioral experiment did not go well, Lucy was prepared with therapy notes that reminded her that she might just need more practice (in therapy sessions) in approaching and talking to people. Had she experienced a negative outcome, her therapist would, at their next session, have elicited and evaluated the conclusions she had drawn, to make sure that Lucy's core beliefs had not been strengthened.

PROBLEMS IN MODIFYING AUTOMATIC THOUGHTS

Difficulties in helping patients change their thinking may arise when patients do not believe their thoughts are distorted and when patients do not experience a decrease in negative affect after evaluating and responding to their thoughts. These two problems are discussed below.

When Patients Do Not Believe Their Thoughts Are Distorted

First, it is important to acknowledge that patients' thoughts may be wholly accurate, and that an important therapeutic goal is for them to learn to assess for themselves the validity and utility of their thoughts. Sometimes it is helpful to give patients a list of cognitive distortions with examples (J. Beck, 1995) and ask them whether any of the thinking errors sound familiar. It may also be useful to ask patients to recall times in the past when their thoughts proved inaccurate. (Most patients, for example, have made anxious predictions that have not come true.)

If patients are convinced of the absolute validity of a thought, despite evidence to the contrary, their automatic thought may also be a core belief. For example, as Hugh lay in bed many mornings, he repeatedly had the thought "I'm a failure." This thought was not specific to just one situation (e.g., "I'm a failure because I don't have a job"). In situation after situation he perceived herself as a failure. Because this cognition was not only an automatic thought but also a rigid, fixed, overgeneralized core belief, it required extensive intervention to change. Hugh's therapist initially labeled the cognition as a belief and helped him to develop a coping response.

THERAPIST: I can see how strong this idea is that you're a failure. In fact, it seems as if it's not just a thought, it's a really deep belief. And it's making you feel so miserable! (*pause*) I wonder if the next time you have this thought you could remind yourself, "No wonder I feel like a failure. I'm depressed. This idea may not be as true as it feels. And therapy can help me get going in my life." (*pause*) Does that sound okay?

HUGH: I could try.

THERAPIST: How about if you write something like that down on a card? How would you like to phrase it?

When Patients Do Not Feel Better After Evaluating and Responding to Their Thinking

Patients may not feel much relief if their therapist did not help them identify automatic thoughts and images that were central to their difficulties. For example, Ann reported that she was very fearful of going to a job interview to be an aide in a day-care center. She and her therapist evaluated her thought: "The interviewer will see how depressed and anxious I am and not hire me." Examining evidence for and against this thought and practicing the interview through role play helped reduce her distress only minimally. Later the therapist found out that Ann had had additional distressing automatic thoughts: "If I get the job, I'll be overwhelmed. I won't know what to do. I'll do things wrong and maybe hurt the children." Ann had also had an image of watching a child under her care fall off a swing and profusely bleed from a head wound. Her anxiety over what could happen on the job outweighed her anxiety about the job interview.

Patients may also not feel better if they change their thinking at an intellectual level, but not at an emotional level. It is often important for therapists to ask patients how much they believe their thought at both levels. Sometimes patients may display this discrepancy in "Yes, but" answers: "*Yes*, I can see that chances are I'll be okay when I go back to work, *but* in my gut, I don't feel that way"; "*Yes*, I can see intellectually that I wasn't such a terrible mother, *but* somehow it still *feels* like I was." Asking patients to engage in a dialogue between their intellectual side and their emotional side can be useful:

THERAPIST: So, you still believe you were a bad mother? What does your gut say?

PATIENT: I should have spent more time with my boys.

THERAPIST: What does your head say?

PATIENT: I did the best I could. I was a single mom, had bills to pay, lots of stress in my life.

THERAPIST: What does your gut say?

PATIENT: Somehow I should have been able to make it different.

THERAPIST: What does your head say?

PATIENT: I don't know.

THERAPIST: Maybe you need to remind yourself what you said before, that in all the important ways you were a fine mother, not a perfect mother, but then no one is, not even your sister. (*pause*) What does your gut say to that?

PATIENT: (*Thinks.*) I don't know. I guess I do believe that.

DYSFUNCTIONAL BELIEFS ABOUT MODIFYING AUTOMATIC THOUGHTS

Patients with challenging problems often hold the same kind of dysfunctional assumptions about modifying their thoughts as those that appear in previous chapters related to setting goals, focusing on a problem, or eliciting their cognitions. These assumptions may, for example, be related to fears of solving problems and getting better ("If I correct my thinking, I'll feel better—but if I feel better, something bad will happen"). Or patients may fear finding out that their thoughts really *are* true. Or they may put a special meaning on finding out that their thoughts are *not* true or not completely true ("If my thoughts are wrong, it means I'm bad or defective").

It is difficult to help patients respond effectively to their automatic thoughts when they cognitively avoid, since significant cognitive change occurs in the presence of negative affect. Therapists often need to use some of the same techniques described in the previous chapter to increase the affect of these patients.

A reluctance to evaluate their thinking may also be related to difficulties in the therapeutic alliance: "If my therapist helps me see that my thoughts are wrong, it means she is superior and I am inferior"; "If my therapist questions the validity of my thoughts, she's invalidating me as a person."

Gordon's therapist noted that Gordon was growing somewhat agitated when she was using Socratic questions to help him evaluate his negative thought that his housemates were looking down at him.

THERAPIST: Gordon, it seems as if this isn't helping very much.

GORDON: No, no, it isn't.

THERAPIST: Can you tell me why it's bothersome?

GORDON: (*Thinks.*) It's like you're telling me I'm wrong.

THERAPIST: I'm sorry if I came across that way. Do you think it would be more helpful if we talked about how you could act around them? How you could show them that they aren't affecting you?

GORDON: Yeah, I guess so.

After practical problem solving, his therapist returned to addressing the process of cognitive restructuring:

THERAPIST: Gordon, let me ask you something. You know, we've talked about how some of your thoughts are 100% true, but, because you're *depressed,* some of your thoughts are not true, or they're not *completely* true. (*pause*) For example, it turned out that it *wasn't* completely true that you couldn't manage around the house. In fact, you do things everyday, *even though you're depressed,* like opening the mail, getting yourself food to eat, washing your dishes. Is that right?

GORDON: (*cautiously*) Yeah.

THERAPIST: And when you realize that you are managing better than you thought, do you feel a little better?

GORDON: Yeah.

THERAPIST: But does it feel bad in some way to find out some of your thinking isn't right?

GORDON: (*Thinks.*) Yeah. (*pause*) You see, my dad was *always* putting me down, always telling me I was wrong. He was so contrary. No matter what I said, he had to take the opposite opinion. If I said it was a nice day out, he'd say, "No, it's going to get too hot." If I said I thought the

Eagles would win the football game, he'd say, "Well, I hope you know they're a lousy team anyway."

THERAPIST: So you could never win.

GORDON: No.

THERAPIST: Well, I'm glad you told me that. Okay, so here's the problem. If I outright agree with everything you tell me, I won't be of much help to you. I'll never help you get over your depression if I agree with you that you're a failure, that you never do anything right.

GORDON: (*Nods.*)

THERAPIST: But when I try to help you figure out whether your depressed thoughts are right or not, it feels bad to you—like I'm telling you you're wrong. Which, in a sense, I guess I *am* doing.

GORDON: Yeah.

THERAPIST: Okay, there are two things I think we can do about this. Can I tell them to you? Then you can see if you think they'll work—or maybe you'll have some ideas, too.

GORDON: Yeah, okay.

THERAPIST: My first thought is, how about if I give you a list of questions for you to ask *yourself* when you have automatic thoughts. Maybe if *you* take the lead in evaluating your thinking, it will feel better.

GORDON: (*slowly*) Okay.

THERAPIST: My second idea is, maybe when you recognize that you're having negative thoughts, you can say to yourself: "Maybe these things aren't completely true. Maybe it's like my father's voice inside my head making me feel bad about myself." (*pause*) Like this thought, "No one in the house wants to have anything to do with me." Does that sound like the kind of put-down your father would have said? Is it possible that the thought isn't completely true?

GORDON: (*Thinks.*) I . . . I'm not sure.

THERAPIST: Well, maybe we could take some more examples that we talked about before. Would your father have looked at your pile of bills and told you what a failure you are? Would he have criticized you for getting a flat tire?

GORDON: Yeah, yeah, he'd say things like that.

THERAPIST: Okay, just to summarize, you may find out that some of your negative thoughts are true—and then we'll do problem solving. But when you find out that some of your thoughts *aren't* true, maybe you can remind yourself that these thoughts are like put-downs from your father and it's *good* to find out that they're wrong.

GORDON: Yeah, I guess so.

Finally, it is not enough to help patients *modify* their distorted thinking: the therapist needs to facilitate their ability to *remember* the new perspective during the rest of the week and into the future. As mentioned previously, it is essential for patients to take home with them therapy notes, cards, or audiotapes containing the most important things they need to remember or do in the coming week.

PROBLEMS IN MODIFYING THOUGHTS BETWEEN SESSIONS

Patients may have difficulty evaluating and responding to their thinking outside of session due to practical problems or interfering cognitions.

Practical Problems

When Patients Experience Significant Distress

As mentioned previously, if the level of patients' negative emotion is too high, they may not be able to evaluate and respond to their thinking. They may need to divert their attention, do relaxation exercises, engage in productive behavior, or talk to other people before their emotion decreases sufficiently to allow them to respond to their thinking effectively.

Patients may not be able to question the validity of their thoughts through tools such as the Dysfunctional Thought Record (J. Beck, 2005), especially initially in therapy, when they are in significant distress. It is far easier for them to read therapy note cards that they and their therapist have devised in the therapy session that contain robust responses to the patient's typical automatic thoughts.

When Standard Tools Are Inappropriate

Worksheets such as the Dysfunctional Thought Record are too complicated for some patients. It may be more useful to give these patients a standard list of questions or perhaps just one or two questions that the therapist judges most likely to be helpful. Candace, a patient with general anxiety disorder and obsessive–compulsive disorder, often predicted dire consequences. She was usually able to reduce her anxiety between sessions by asking herself, "What's the best thing that could happen? What's the most realistic outcome?" It was most helpful for Howard to ask himself, "Is it possible that this thought is not completely true?" James did best when asking himself, "If my brother had this thought, what would I tell him?" Dolores often felt better when she asked herself, "What would [my therapist] probably say about this?"

Another problem can arise with some patients whose thinking is obsessive. Rather than use tools such as the Dysfunctional Thought

Record, patients may need to label their thoughts as "obsessive" and carry on with their activities, instead of trying to modify their thinking. Dena continually had obsessive thoughts when she had to make even unimportant decisions about what clothes to wear, what food to buy, what social plans to make, what shopping to do. It proved to be of limited use for her to respond to her thought "It will be bad if I [make a wrong decision]." It was far more useful for her to learn to say: "That's just another obsessive thought. I don't have to pay too much attention to it. It's making me think that this decision is life or death, which it isn't. I should just make the decision on a practical basis—like what is easiest for me to do."

When Patients' Expectations Are Too High

Sometimes patients do a reasonable job of responding to their automatic thoughts between sessions but they do not realize it—because they expect that they should be able to *eliminate* their negative emotions. A good guideline is that even a 10% reduction in their distress means the process of responding to their thoughts was worthwhile. (Of course, many patients find their negative emotions reduce much more than that.) Patients also need to know that it may take significant work over a period of time to change automatic thoughts that are closely tied to beliefs.

THERAPIST: You know, Joe, I'm not surprised that you still believe everyday that you aren't doing enough. After all, in the past year alone, how many times a day have you told yourself that?

JOE: Lots.

THERAPIST: Maybe dozens of times a day, everyday? So it's going to take a while for you really to consider that maybe what you're doing *is* reasonable and *is* enough.

Interfering Thoughts

Sometimes patients resist trying to modify or respond to their automatic thoughts at home due to their dysfunctional ideas. Many of these ideas were described under "homework" in Chapter 9. In the following transcript the therapist probes for interfering thoughts and helps the patient respond to them.

THERAPIST: So when you had all those negative thoughts this week, did you think of trying to answer them back?

PATIENT: Yeah, but it just seemed too hard. I didn't want to do it. I just wanted to go to sleep and feel all better when I got up.

THERAPIST: Were you able to do that? Did you fall asleep? Did you feel all better when you woke up?

PATIENT: No, I still felt lousy.

THERAPIST: Looking back, do you think you would have been better off or worse off reading the therapy notes we wrote together?

PATIENT: I don't know.

THERAPIST: Do you have them here? [If not, the therapist can give the patient his/her copy.] Can you read them out loud now?

After the patient reads the notes aloud the therapist asks:

THERAPIST: So what do you think? *If* you had been able to read them and *if* you had believed them, would you have felt better, worse, or the same?

PATIENT: Well, the same or better, I guess. Not worse.

THERAPIST: Can we talk about how you can get yourself to read them this week, then?

PATIENT: Okay.

THERAPIST: Can you imagine that it's after dinner tonight and you know you're supposed to read the cards? What goes through your mind?

The following are other typical thoughts that might get in the way of patients responding to their automatic thoughts at home. Therapists can discuss these thoughts with patients and help them create (idiosyncratically composed) therapy notes such as the following:

Interfering thought: I shouldn't have to work so hard at this.

Response: I wish I didn't have to do this, but not doing it has pretty much kept me stuck. I'm probably overestimating how hard it will be to do it [read my therapy notes or do a Dysfunctional Thought Record]. I can tolerate trying it for a couple of minutes.

Interfering thought: My therapist should fix me.

Response: I know in my heart of hearts that she can't fix me, that I'm only going to get better if *I* make a strong effort.

Interfering thought: I'm too helpless/incompetent to affect my mood.

Response: I have been able to affect my mood sometimes in the past. I won't actually know whether I can help myself feel better right now until I try. The worst that will happen is that [responding to my thoughts] won't help at all. It's worth the risk to try.

USING AND VARYING STANDARD STRATEGIES
TO MODIFY SPONTANEOUS IMAGES

As noted in the previous chapter, patients often experience three types of images: automatic thought level images, metaphorical images, and images in the form of memories. Various techniques, described extensively in *Cognitive Therapy: Basics and Beyond* (J. Beck, 1995), can be used to help patients modify their images or the meaning of their images. Some of these techniques are presented below.

Automatic Thought Level Images

While images can be reality-tested through standard Socratic questioning, patients often experience additional relief when they learn to change the image, follow the image through to a safe conclusion, or see themselves coping with the misfortune they imagine has befallen them.

Changing the Image

Randy, described briefly in the previous chapter, was highly anxious when he had thoughts and an image of being fired. His distress decreased when his therapist helped him examine the validity of his thoughts and he recognized that although he had missed some deadlines at work, he had overall performed adequately. His anxiety decreased even more significantly, however, when his therapist helped him change his image. He had initially envisioned his boss calling him into his office, sharply criticizing his work performance, and telling him to leave the building and never return. His therapist helped him envision a more realistic image of his boss reviewing his evaluation with him, pointing out positive aspects of his work performance, and telling him what he needed to improve.

Continuing the Image in a More Positive Way

Justin had a spontaneous image of becoming highly anxious as he walked along a busy city street, having a panic attack, and fainting. His therapist asked him questions to help him continue the image until he was in a safer place.

THERAPIST: Okay, so can you see yourself lying on the ground? (*pause*) What would you like to imagine happens next?

JUSTIN: I'm not sure.

THERAPIST: Well, would you like to imagine that someone comes over to help?

JUSTIN: (*Nods.*)

THERAPIST: Would you like it to be a man or a woman?

JUSTIN: A woman, I think.

THERAPIST: Okay, can you see her crouching down beside you? What does she say?

JUSTIN: I guess she says, "Oh, are you all right? Can I help you?"

THERAPIST: And what do you say?

JUSTIN: I don't know.

THERAPIST: Well, would you like to imagine yourself getting up and saying, "I think I'm okay. But could you help me find a place to sit down?"

JUSTIN: Yeah, that sounds good.

THERAPIST: And where do you want to imagine she takes you? Someplace close by?

JUSTIN: Someplace not too crowded. (*Thinks.*) Maybe the lobby of an office building.

THERAPIST: Can you see her helping you get up? Can you see her leading you into the office building? What happens next?

The therapist continues facilitating this extension of Justin's image until he is feeling much calmer; in this case, Justin imagines himself going into the office building and sitting on a bench. The solicitous woman brings him a glass of water. Then Justin drives home, goes into the living room, and watches the news on television. By that point, he imagines that his anxiety is almost completely gone.

Imagining Coping with What Has Happened

Brian's mother was quite ill and he felt quite distressed when he imagined himself alone by his mother's bedside as she died. His therapist helped him imagine a more realistic scene. He saw his family entering the room to comfort him. Then he saw himself talking to a nurse to find out what he had to do next. He imagined calling his best friend, whose father had recently died, to ask about funeral parlors and to find out what else he had to do that day. Then the therapist had him jump ahead in time, imagining the funeral. She asked him to describe what was happening, what he was thinking, and what he was feeling. He realized that it would be excruciatingly painful but that he would get through the experience. Then his therapist asked him to imagine himself 6 months later. Brian saw himself back to life as usual, feeling grief, but not the high degree of pain he had previously felt. Seeing himself coping with the very difficult experience of his mother's death diminished Brian's immediate feelings of devastation considerably.

Metaphorical Images

When patients make metaphorical statements, it is often helpful to ask them for an image and help them change the image in some way. At one point in therapy, Mitchell reported that he was feeling more hopeless, as if he were running into a brick wall. His therapist asked him to describe what the wall looked like. She then asked him how he could deal with this obstacle: how could he go over, under, around, or through the wall. Mitchell replied that he would need a sledgehammer to break through. His therapist discussed with him what the sledgehammer represented—and helped him see that perhaps it was a tool he was creating in treatment. Since he had had only a few sessions of therapy, perhaps the skills he had learned amounted to a child's small wooden hammer. However, he could learn more skills week by week, until the hammer would morph into a large sledgehammer. When Mitchell imagined himself breaking through the wall with the sledgehammer, he felt a sense of relief and his hopelessness decreased.

Therapists can often use images to extend a negative metaphorical representation in a positive direction. Carla became highly distressed at times, especially when she had the thought "I'm drowning," which was accompanied by an image of herself sinking below the surface of a deep lake. Her therapist helped her envision a lifeboat filled with all the people in her current support network rescuing her and later teaching her how to swim. Using metaphors to modify beliefs is further illustrated in Chapter 13.

Extending a Memory

Distressing memories are often comprised of a discrete event at one point of time. Patients remember what was happening while they felt the most upset but their spontaneous memories usually do not include the time following this event—a time when they have survived and are feeling less pain.

Kay sometimes had a disturbing memory about something that had happened to her at school one day when she was 8 years old. A group of girls on the playground taunted her about her clothes and her "stupid accent." Kay had felt humiliated. Spontaneously recalling this event in visual form, she imaged only the upsetting event itself. Her quick image did *not* include the relatively more positive immediate aftermath: she returned to the classroom, focused on her schoolwork, and then went home to watch television. In the future, in fact, this group of girls just ignored her. Several years later, she worked on the middle school newsletter with one of them and actually became friendly with her. This memory caused her a great deal of distress until her therapist coached her to remember what had happened immediately following the event and later on.

When Teresa was discussing her fear that she would not survive if her husband died, she too reported a memory of a particular moment in time, when she had tried to stay alone overnight for the first time in her life. She had been so frightened that she had left her new apartment after midnight and returned home. Her therapist helped her recall the bigger picture, that eventually she had moved to an apartment for a period of time with a friend and, though she never liked the experience, was able to spend several weekends alone when her roommate went out of town.

SUMMARY

Patients may have difficulty modifying their automatic thoughts in session for a variety of reasons. When asking standard Socratic questions is insufficient, therapists often need to use different kinds of questions and techniques and ascertain whether patients may have beliefs that interfere with the process of examining their thoughts. Therapists also need to ascertain whether patients experience difficulty modifying their thoughts for homework and, as with other problems, specify and remediate the difficulty. Special imaginal techniques are useful in helping patients respond to their distressing images.

CHAPTER 12

Challenges in Modifying Assumptions

Some assumptions of patients with challenging problems are relatively easy to modify, especially those that are situation-specific. These assumptions are really at the automatic thought level and are usually predictive in nature. Assumptions at an intermediate belief level are more difficult to modify and are the primary focus of this chapter. They are broader, more strongly held, and usually incorporate a coping strategy or reflect a core belief. The first section of this chapter differentiates these two groups of assumptions. The next section describes using and varying standard strategies to modify intermediate belief level assumptions, and outlines dysfunctional beliefs that interfere with modifying assumptions. Finally, interventions for three dysfunctional assumptions that often interfere with treatment are illustrated through a lengthy case example.

DIFFERENTIATING AUTOMATIC THOUGHT LEVEL ASSUMPTIONS FROM INTERMEDIATE BELIEF LEVEL ASSUMPTIONS

Some assumptions are actually automatic thoughts that pop up in patients' minds in specific situations. Therapists often work on these predictive assumptions first, before working on the broader assumption with which they are associated. For example, Audrey, a patient with avoidant personality disorder, had the following automatic thoughts in an assumption form:

> "If I ask my roommate to turn down the music, she'll get angry."
> "If I ask for help at [the clothing store], the clerks will get annoyed."
> "If I ask [my coworker] to cover the phones for me, she'll refuse."

Her therapist used standard strategies discussed in Chapter 11 to help Audrey evaluate these predictive assumptions, then suggested that she try some behavioral experiments to test them directly. Following these successful behavioral experiments, they derived and evaluated a broader assumption, which was at the intermediate belief level:

"If I express my needs or desires, people will feel put-upon and refuse me."

Audrey had never put this idea into words before. This assumption did not pop into her mind in specific situations. Rather it reflected a general understanding. Deeper level assumptions such as this one are usually more rigid and generalized than automatic thought level assumptions. These intermediate level assumptions may be predictive or meaning-related.

Heidi, for example, held the following intermediate level *predictive* assumption:

"If I'm not a 'Supermom,' my kids won't do well in life."

She also had the following *meaning-related* assumptions:

"If my kids are unhappy, it means I've done something wrong."
"If I'm not doing things perfectly, I'm a bad mother."

USING AND VARYING STANDARD STRATEGIES
TO MODIFY ASSUMPTIONS

Therapists use the same kinds of techniques to modify assumptions as they use to modify automatic thoughts. They include:

- Educating patients about assumptions.
- Using Socratic questioning.
- Examining the advantages and disadvantages of believing an assumption.
- Devising behavioral experiments.
- Acting "as if."
- Creating a cognitive continuum.
- Formulating a more functional assumption.
- Doing rational-emotional role plays.
- Using imaginal techniques.
- Using metaphors.
- Questioning others about their assumptions.
- Examining the childhood origin of assumptions.

Many of these techniques and their variations are described in the extended case example that follows, in the context of modifying three key assumptions that interfere with treatment:

1. "If I let myself feel bad, I'll fall apart (I'll be overwhelmed, I won't be able to stand it, I won't be able to function, I'll be miserable forever, I'll go crazy)."
2. "If I try to solve problems, I'll fail."
3. "If I get better (through therapy), my life will get worse."

Sometimes assumptions such as these are so strongly held that the therapist needs to help the patient modify them before the patient is willing to engage in treatment. In the case example below, the therapist identified these assumptions early in treatment and started to help the patient modify them. Unlike most patients, Helen required extensive work, using many therapeutic strategies, to modify her assumptions, particularly the first one. The patient was able—slowly and over time—to increase her commitment to working in therapy. They continued to work on these assumptions throughout the course of treatment.

EXTENDED CASE EXAMPLE

Helen was a 30-year-old woman who had been chronically depressed and anxious since her early 20s. She had been intermittently employed as a clerk in various retail stores. Her father, an alcoholic, had been physically abusive to her as she was growing up. Her mother, depressed herself, was quite isolative, inattentive to her and her sister, and emotionally distant. At the beginning of treatment, Helen's functioning was low: she was unemployed, slept much of the day, and watched television most of the night. She left home primarily to do errands, go to her friend's house, or help out her sister. Her apartment was a mess; she was behind in paying bills. Some days she did not even get dressed. Before she began cognitive therapy treatment, her anxiety had been low, primarily due to her extensive avoidance. Helen related a long history of seeing mental health professionals.

The three assumptions listed in the section above significantly interfered with Helen's ability to engage in treatment. She arrived late to sessions and resisted setting goals, responding to her cognitions, and doing homework assignments. Although interventions for the three assumptions are presented separately in the following discussion, in actuality her therapist usually addressed more than one assumption in each session, in the context of setting agendas, setting and reviewing homework, and doing problem solving. To overcome Helen's avoidance of homework, for example, her therapist had to work on all three assumptions. He made dozens of interventions over time to modify her dysfunctional assumptions and to help her develop and strengthen new, more functional assumptions. She slowly made progress and was able to successfully terminate therapy after a year of treatment.

Assumption 1: "If I Feel Bad, I'll Fall Apart (but If I Avoid Feeling Bad, I'll Be Okay)."

This assumption accounted in large part for how limited Helen's life was. She avoided thinking about things that distressed her and she avoided engaging in behavior that she predicted would lead to her feeling anxious or depressed. There was, in fact, some evidence in support of this assumption. The "best" period in her life, her late teens, was followed by the "worst" period in her life when a boyfriend ("the one and only perfect guy" for her) rejected her. Over the course of the next few months, she fell into a deep depression, attempted suicide, and was hospitalized. Her level of depression eventually decreased but never fully remitted. Helen also became alcohol-dependent, trying to deaden her negative emotions with which she believed she could not cope. Several years before she started treatment with her cognitive therapist, she had gained full remission from her alcohol dependence with the help of several rounds of rehab and therapy. After that, her primary strategy to avoid experiencing negative emotion was to engage in significant cognitive and behavioral avoidance. When she did feel upset, she used distractions such as watching television or eating.

Helen's therapist first collected evidence of this assumption in the second session, when Helen reported that she had not done any therapy homework during the previous week. When asked about her automatic thoughts when she was thinking about doing her assignment, Helen reported that she was worried that reading a booklet on depression might make her feel worse, not better. She had considered doing the second part of the homework—getting out of her apartment more, but again reported that she had become worried that she would feel too anxious. At the following session, Helen had again not done her (significantly scaled back) homework assignment for the same reason. Her therapist asked her to complete the second part of a conditional assumption.

THERAPIST: Helen, how would you answer this: "If I do things that could make me feel bad, then 'blank' could happen?" What's your biggest concern?

HELEN: That (*pause*) I'd just . . . fall apart.

THERAPIST: How much do you believe that?

HELEN: I don't know . . . . A lot. I just feel like I'm on the brink a lot of the time.

THERAPIST: Well, no wonder you don't want to do these things for homework.

Collecting Current Data about the Assumption

Later in the session and in the next few sessions, the therapist collected more information about Helen's assumption:

Determining the Degree of Belief in the Assumption

- "How much do you believe this idea right now, 'If I feel bad, I could fall apart'?"
- "How much do you believe it intellectually, and how much do you believe it emotionally?"

Defining Terms

- "What does 'fall apart' mean? What does it look like?"

Assessing the Worst Fear

- "Are you afraid anything worse than 'falling apart' could happen to you—or is falling apart the worst?"

Assessing the Predicted Aftermath

- "If you did fall apart, how long are you afraid it would last?"
- "What are you afraid would happen next?"
- (*Probing for an image*) "What would that look like?"

Assessing Coping Strategies

- "What could you do to pull yourself together faster?"

Assessing the Pervasiveness of the Assumption

- "In which situations do you have this idea?"
- "In which situations do you *not* have this idea?"

Assessing the Pervasiveness of Maladaptive Coping Strategies

- "Which situations do you avoid so you won't feel bad?"

Assessing Safety Behaviors

- "What do you do in situations you *do* have to enter—or when you have to do things that could make you feel bad—so you don't fall apart?"

Developing a More Realistic Belief

Helen's therapist reviewed much of the data he had collected thus far to help Helen consider a more adaptive and valid viewpoint. He frequently checked how much she believed this new belief in the context of reviewing her experiences in the preceding week, her homework, and the problems she had put on the agenda.

Presenting a New Belief

■ "Based on what we've talked about so far, would you think it's a little more accurate to say that if you feel bad, you'll hate the feeling but won't fall apart?"

Assessing the Strength of the New Belief

■ "How much do you believe this new idea, intellectually and emotionally?"

Collecting Ongoing Data about the Assumption

Helen's therapist continually asked her to rate (at both an intellectual and an emotional level) how strongly she still believed she would fall apart if she engaged in specific feared activities and how strongly she believed that she might "feel" as if she were falling apart, though in actuality she would be anxious but okay. They also collected evidence contrary to her dysfunctional assumption and supportive of her new assumption, listing situations in which she had felt distressed but had not fallen apart. Additionally they collected and reframed evidence that seemed to support her dysfunctional assumption.

Helen's therapist continually asked her what still made her believe that her assumption was true, then helped her reframe each piece of evidence. For example, Helen went to the drugstore to pick up two prescriptions. Although she was very nervous, she was able to ask the pharmacist an important question. When she got home, she realized that the pharmacist had given her just one of the medications. She returned to the pharmacy but left without asking about her second medication. Her therapist helped her see that going in the first place was a successful experience and that her decision not to talk to the pharmacist on her second trip there did not confirm that high anxiety would make her fall apart—it only confirmed that she *believed* that high anxiety would make her fall apart.

Setting Up a Therapeutic Hypothesis

When Helen claimed she had not fallen apart because she either avoided situations or used safety behaviors, her therapist suggested the following hypothesis:

> ■ "I guess there are two possibilities of what would have happened if you *hadn't* avoided the situation or used safety behaviors. Either your anxiety would have gotten worse and you *would* have fallen apart. Or, even though you *felt* like you were close to falling apart, you really weren't—and, in fact, anxiety *doesn't* make you fall apart."

Presenting the Treatment Plan

When Helen's therapist started teaching her techniques to use when she was anxious, he was careful to distinguish between coping with negative emotion and tolerating it:

> ■ "Helen, the first step in treatment is going to be to teach you skills to cope with your anxiety instead of avoiding it. Ultimately, though, it's going to be important for you to prove to yourself over and over that you can just tolerate it. And so at some point we'll actually have you *not* use these new skills, so you can get over your fear of getting anxious once and for all."

Doing Behavioral Tests during Sessions

Helen initially tried to avoid discussing problems she predicted would lead her to feel too anxious, such as finding a job or going to social events. She agreed to a behavioral test and indeed found that while she was mildly anxious discussing these topics, she did not become overly anxious. Her therapist framed Helen's subsequent anxiety-provoking experiences during sessions as behavioral tests (that always disconfirmed her assumption).

Examining Advantages and Disadvantages of the Dysfunctional Assumption

As a result of their discussion, Helen and her therapist devised the following chart, which listed the disadvantages of the belief and the advantages of the belief—with a reframe (alternative perspective) for each advantage.

Disadvantages of Believing I'll Fall Apart	Advantages of Believing I'll Fall Apart (with Reframes)
• My life will stay lousy. • I'll keep on being depressed. • I won't get a job. • I won't have much money. • I won't get a boyfriend. • I'll have lots of anxiety when I'm forced to do things. • I won't feel good about myself.	• I can continue to avoid *but* avoidance brings me relief only in the short run and I feel bad in the long run. • I won't have to take risks *but* most of the things I'm avoiding are low risk anyway and my therapist can help me with the others. • I can maintain the status quo *but* the status quo is keeping me depressed.

Providing Psychoeducation

Helen's therapist drew a chart to help himself and Helen understand why her avoidance was so pervasive (Figure 12.1). Depicting her typical avoidance scenario in this way helped Helen to see why her pattern of avoidance was so entrenched (due to an immediate cessation of anxiety and an immediate feeling of relief). However, it also reminded her of the highly

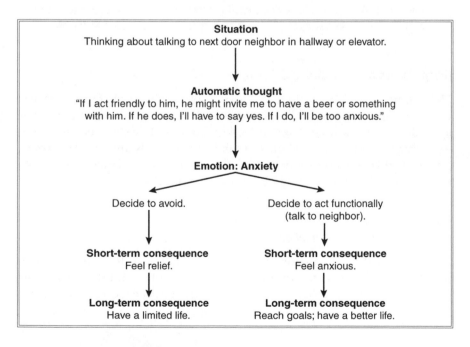

FIGURE 12.1. Helen's avoidance scenario.

undesirable long-term consequences of her avoidance and the highly *desirable* long-term consequences of tolerating her anxiety and refraining from avoidance behavior.

Helen's therapist also used a diagram to help her see that her avoidance, instead of ridding herself of anxiety, actually helped keep her anxiety going.

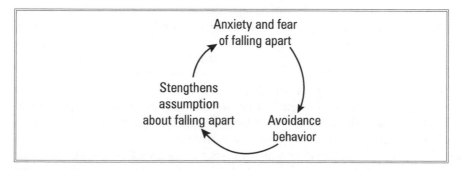

Her therapist continually prompted Helen to remember that her fear of falling apart was based on a time when she felt *hopeless* and *depressed*, not necessarily anxious.

Seeking Alternative Explanations for (Avoidance) Behavior

They also discussed other reasons Helen had for not doing things. As it turned out, sometimes Helen avoided activities for fear she would immediately feel bad; sometimes it was because she did not *want* to do things; sometimes she feared she would do things poorly; and sometimes she feared that doing things *now* would mean she'd have to take on greater challenges in the *future*. (Interventions to address these fears are presented later in this chapter.)

Using Imagery

Helen's therapist used imagery techniques with her. Among other things, he induced coping imagery, asking Helen to imagine herself engaging in specific feared activities, feeling anxious, but then feeling better after she had used the anxiety management techniques she had learned in treatment.

Identifying/Modifying Cognitive Distortions

Having identified Helen's dysfunctional thoughts, her therapist helped her learn to label the cognitive errors she was making in order to respond to her thoughts more effectively. For example, Helen displayed a lot of dichotomous thinking. She and her therapist discussed the all-or-nothing nature of her view of emotion ("Either I feel calm and in control [of my emotions] or I feel terrible and am in danger of falling apart").

Modifying Homework

Helen failed to do any homework during the first 2 weeks of treatment. She and her therapist collaboratively agreed to scale back Helen's assignments significantly. At their third session, rather than setting an assignment to change her behavior, her therapist suggested she just think about engaging in adaptive behavior and monitor her thinking. Helen's dysfunctional assumption about experiencing negative emotion quickly became apparent. Her next assignment (which she continued for several months) was to report to the therapist situations she had encountered during the week in which she felt distressed but did not fall apart. Two weeks later, Helen agreed to "easy" behavioral assignments.

Reading therapy notes was an essential part of homework. Initially, Helen just read cards with conclusions she had drawn in session. For example, an initial coping card designed to respond to her negative assumptions about experiencing distress read:

> I have an idea that if I start to feel bad, I'll fall apart. But I've felt bad thousands of times just in the past few years and I didn't fall apart. I was in an entirely different situation when I did end up in the hospital.

Initially Helen read her coping cards only two or three times a week but she shortly began reading them almost daily.

Doing Behavioral Experiments

Helen did literally dozens and dozens of behavioral experiments for homework to test her assumption, starting at a very easy level (e.g., going through her mail for just 10 minutes, asking for information at the library). Coping cards helped motivate her:

> Doing this may make me feel a little bad, but I can stand it. It won't make me fall apart. I've done lots of other things in the past few months that were *more* distressing and I didn't fall apart.

Reading a coping card *after* testing her assumption was also important:

> I tolerated the anxiety and I didn't fall apart.
>
> Maybe my predictions just aren't true.
>
> I deserve a lot of credit for doing this.

Making the behavioral experiments quite easy greatly increased the probability that Helen would follow through with them. Another important initial intervention was to allow—indeed to encourage—Helen to use anxiety management strategies to reduce her distress. Another card, devised early in treatment, reminded her of what she could do:

When I Feel Bad: Things to Do

- Read my therapy notes.
- Call Jean, Annette.
- Go for a walk.
- Bake bread.
- Look for new humor websites.
- Do relaxation exercises.
- Do a DTR [Dysfunctional Thought Record] in my head.
- *Or* I can sit with it; see that I don't fall apart; see how long it lasts.

Her therapist indicated, however, that it would be important for Helen to fully experience distress, without engaging in any of these behaviors, so she could fully test her assumption about falling apart and so she could learn to tolerate negative emotion. A coping card helped her remember this:

Using [these techniques] can help me feel more comfortable. But I don't need to, because feeling bad does not lead to falling apart.

General therapy notes helped Helen carry through with behavioral experiments. Specific coping cards helped her work her way through a hierarchy of situations she had avoided for fear of experiencing too much distress. For example, Helen had procrastinated about calling a doctor to discuss a problem with allergies that had become significantly worse. She predicted that she would feel too uncomfortable being scrutinized by the doctor, nurse, office personnel, and other patients. Her therapist discussed her automatic thoughts about this situation at length. The conclusions Helen drew (see below) served as a model for many other behavioral experiments she did later.

If I Feel Like Avoiding Calling the Doctor

Remember I had predicted I would feel too anxious before my first [cognitive] therapy appointment but it turned out okay and I have lots more coping techniques now than I did before. Even if I do feel uncomfortable, I won't fall apart. I can stand it. I'll probably feel the most uncomfortable just before the appointment and for the first few minutes, but then I'll probably feel a little better. I can make myself feel worse by focusing on how bad I feel or better by looking around to see what is really happening. The people who work there will be focusing on their jobs—and will not be evaluating me as a person. Other patients may look up when I come in the room but probably only momentarily.

At every session her therapist praised Helen for completing her homework and positively reinforced her new learning. He helped her recognize that her predictions about falling apart were incorrect. He frequently asked, "What does this experience tell you about your ability to handle feeling bad?"

Decreasing Safety Behaviors

As Helen eroded the degree of belief in her dysfunctional assumption, her therapist helped her identify behaviors she was still engaging in to reduce her distress. While much of her avoidance was quite apparent, some of it was more subtle, such as walking with her head down so she wouldn't see neighbors when she took a walk or not making eye contact with store clerks. He encouraged her to do behavioral experiments in which she refrained from using safety behaviors.

Historically Based Interventions

The techniques described above primarily focused on examining Helen's assumption as it became activated in current situations. It was also helpful for Helen to review her history, to determine when and how she had started to develop this assumption, to find data contrary to her assumption, and to reframe the meaning of past events related to the assumption.

> ■ "How long have you had this idea? When do you think it first developed?"
> ■ "In which situations did you actually fall apart and how long did you stay fallen apart?"
> ■ "How did you get over the experience?"

The therapist also asked Helen to recall times throughout her life when she was upset but did not completely fall apart. She eventually compiled a list that was over three pages long.

Recognizing the Childhood Origin of the Dysfunctional Assumption

It was useful for Helen to recognize that some of her fear of experiencing negative emotion originated when she was a child. She had memories of feeling overcome with sadness and anxiety when her parents (frequently and loudly) argued, when she anticipated that her father *might* abuse her or her sister, and when her drunken father *did* hurt her physically. Her therapist helped her realize that at the time she really did not have coping tools for dealing with the extreme emotion she felt. On the other hand, she had not fallen apart.

Using Imagery to Gain a Wider Perspective

Helen sometimes had a memory of the day she was hospitalized, when she was in abject emotional pain. The therapist helped her recognize that this image was like a "sound-bite" in time—it neglected to include the period leading up to her hospitalization and the period after her hospitalization as she slowly recovered. She was able to recall that she did not suddenly fall apart (her current fear). Rather she went downhill over the course of many weeks, and eventually she did feel much less pain, even if her depression did not lift entirely.

Next her therapist had her recall in imagery her gradual improvement during hospitalization and reexperience the relief she felt when she went home. He also had her visualize in detail a typical day 6 months after the hospitalization when she was back at work and interacting with her family.

Assumption 2: "If I Have a Problem, I Won't Be Able to Solve It (but If I Ignore It or Avoid It, I'll Be Okay)."

Helen's therapist uncovered this assumption early in treatment when Helen resisted setting goals and naming problems for the agenda. Helen had some evidence that this assumption was valid. She generally avoided problem solving, gave up prematurely, or relied on others to help her with her difficulties. She was particularly deficient in skills to solve interpersonal problems. When she quarreled with others, she withdrew (e.g., quit jobs, unilaterally ended therapy with previous therapists, stopped contacting friends, refused to see her father).

Having identified this important assumption, Helen's therapist used the techniques listed below to help her reframe her thinking:

- Collecting current and historical data to identify the origin, pervasiveness, frequency, and strength of the belief over time.
- Discussing the *meaning* to Helen of trying to solve problems and failing ("It shows how incompetent I am"); identifying alternative reasons for failing to solve problems; reframing negative outcomes as demonstrating specific skill deficits rather than global defects.
- Discussing advantages and disadvantages of the assumption and reframing the advantages.
- Summarizing relevant childhood experiences to normalize the development of the belief; predicting how Helen might have behaved differently through time had she not held this assumption ("If you had not believed that you were incapable and couldn't solve problems, what might you have done when [you were struggling in school]?").

- Developing a more functional belief.
- Doing rational-emotional role plays (see pp. 292–295), first with the therapist, then with herself, to elicit and then respond to evidence Helen still used to support the assumption.
- Reviewing and drawing conclusions about Helen's current and past *positive* experiences with problem solving ("What does this tell you about your ability to solve problems? What does this say about you?"). She recorded her conclusions on cards:

I *assume* if I have a problem, I won't be able to solve it. But this is an idea, not necessarily a truth. As long as I keep telling myself that, I'll stay stuck, not even try to solve problems, and my life will continue to be lousy. If I had believed I *could* solve problems, I might have come up with ideas such as applying for tuition money for the training program or getting a better apartment.

If I try to solve a problem and fail, what's the big deal? It doesn't mean I'm incompetent. The problem may be out of my control (e.g., how Dad treats Mom). At worst it means I couldn't do a *specific* thing well enough (like convincing my landlord to repaint the apartment). I can always talk about that kind of problem in therapy.

When I think I can't solve a problem, see if it's more true that I just don't *want to try*, rather than that I will definitely not be able to solve it.

When I was growing up, I started to believe that I couldn't solve problems, but that wasn't completely true even then. What is true is that I couldn't change dad's behavior. But I did solve other problems everyday, like dealing with my sister, getting through school, and so on.

Also I didn't have role models who solved problems—Mom and Dad avoided solving problems, too.

No wonder I grew up with this belief.

When I think today that I can't solve problems, remind myself that this is an idea left over from childhood and it may or may not apply to this problem I'm currently facing.

Assumption 3: "If I Get Better, My Life Will Get Worse (but If I Stay as I Am, at Least I Can Maintain the Status Quo)."

This third assumption was related to the first two. Helen was afraid that if she improved she would have to face challenges so distressing she would would fail and then fall apart. Getting better meant to her that she would have to take risks, make herself vulnerable, expose her incompetence, and feel terrible. It also meant that she would no longer be able to depend on her therapist, her sister, and her friend Jean. She displayed dichotomous thinking:

"Either I'm mentally unhealthy and can't be expected to get a job or act functionally—and so it's legitimate to depend on other people. Or I'm mentally healthy and I have to act completely functionally, completely on my own—which I know I can't do."

Her therapist again made many interventions over time—for example, by collecting current and historical data about the assumption, monitoring the strength of the assumption on an ongoing basis, collecting evidence contrary to the assumption, reframing evidence that seemed to support the assumption, developing a new assumption, and determining how and why she first developed the assumption. Other key interventions included the following:

Using Imagery

Helen's therapist asked what she feared her life would look like if indeed she improved in treatment and her life got worse. She reported two spontaneous images that seemed to encapsulate her fears. In the first image, she saw herself feeling overwhelmed while trying to take inventory at a store. She saw her supervisor yelling at her while her coworkers smirked. In the image she felt highly anxious, embarrassed, and humiliated, and saw herself as a complete failure and object of ridicule. In a second image, she saw herself at a social gathering, isolated in a corner, unable to break into a conversation, feeling defective and anxious. Both of these images had elements of real-life situations she had experienced in the past.

Helen's therapist helped her modify the images. She visualized in detail working in a small shop, for a boss who was a reasonable human being. Later in treatment, he had her imagine herself being assertive if she *did* have an unreasonable boss and quitting if the situation became intolerable. He also had her imagine walking into a social gathering, feeling nervous at first, but bravely introducing herself to someone she saw standing alone. She saw herself making small talk, feeling nervous at first, but gradually becoming more comfortable.

Decatastrophizing

As he had done previously, Helen's therapist helped her see that she would not necessarily *have* to take on big challenges once she felt better. She would have the *choice* of doing so or not.

Increasing Resources

Helen and her therapist also discussed the resources she would have before tackling a big challenge. She was learning new skills in therapy to counter her sabotaging thoughts, to decrease her distress, to help her face avoided tasks, and to make her life in general more fulfilling. She would always have an escape hatch; she could, for example, quit a job if she had to or call on Jean, her sister, or her therapist.

Graded Exposure to Challenges

Helen's therapist also had her recognize that before she was ready to face significant challenges, she would have mastered easier ones. He drew a staircase to illustrate this idea (see p. 267) and asked Helen to help her figure out the intermediate steps she would take before getting a job. Helen's therapist helped her see that whenever she thought about getting a job, she pictured herself having to make a huge jump from the bottom of the staircase to the top. She felt much better when her therapist showed her that she would take just one step at a time. He also reassured her that they could make half-steps or quarter-steps if it turned out the steps they had initially devised turned out to be too big.

SUMMARY

Modifying broad intermediate level assumptions is more difficult than modifying situation specific automatic thoughts or assumptions at the automatic thought level. Therapists use many of the same techniques in modifying assumptions that they use in modifying automatic thoughts and face many of the same challenges. Using a variety of strategies over time is often necessary. Follow-up and maintenance are important to ensure that patients apply what they have learned in therapy in the presence of new stressors that may threaten to reactivate their old assumptions.

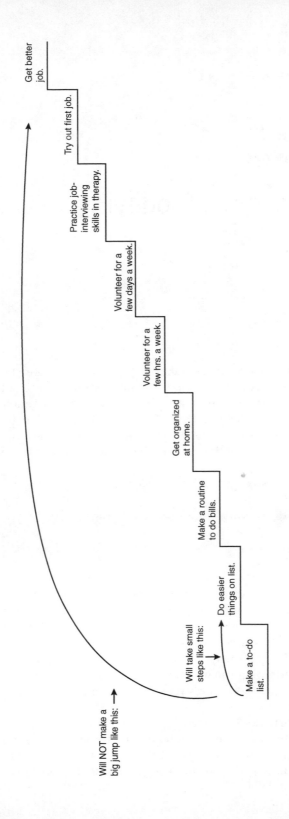

Will NOT make a big jump like this: →

Will take small steps like this: →

Get better job.

Try out first job.

Practice job-interviewing skills in therapy.

Volunteer for a few days a week.

Volunteer for a few hrs. a week.

Get organized at home.

Make a routine to do bills.

Do easier things on list.

Make a to-do list.

CHAPTER 13

Challenges in Modifying Core Beliefs

Modification of core beliefs takes a great deal of consistent hard work over many months of treatment for many patients with challenging problems. It is important to have a realistic sense of how much patients can modify their core beliefs. Patients are unlikely to change their beliefs entirely; in fact, most people have helpless or unlovable beliefs that become activated from time to time. Therapeutic goals are for patients to:

- Erode the strength of core beliefs and reduce the frequency of their activation.
- Reduce distress and think and behave more adaptively when beliefs are activated.
- Develop and strengthen more realistic, more functional beliefs.

Therapists need to consider carefully when to start evaluating core beliefs. Therapy would be greatly speeded up if therapists could help patients change their core beliefs at the first session, but most patients hold these beliefs much too strongly to change them so easily. Early in treatment, therapists may start hypothesizing about patients' core beliefs, through ascertaining the meaning of their automatic thoughts (see Chapter 9). They may assess the strength of these beliefs and try some belief modification.

When patients have challenging problems, though, therapists may find their efforts initially unsuccessful. Core beliefs are often more easily modified toward the middle part of therapy, when patients are less symptomatic and have had many positive experiences of testing and modifying their automatic thoughts and assumptions. Having discovered other cognitions were inaccurate and recognizing that changing their cognitions leads to an improved reaction, patients are then usually willing to consider that their core beliefs may also be inaccurate and may be willing to do the hard work to evaluate and modify them.

By the middle of therapy, the therapeutic alliance is also stronger. It is important for therapists to appreciate just how vulnerable and anxious some patients feel when they engage in the process of questioning beliefs that are integral to their sense of self. Although Helen (described in the previous chapter) did not like believing that she was defective, she began to become quite distressed when her therapist started to help her question that belief. She expressed her fear outright: "If I'm not defective, who am I?"

In a sense, though, therapists are indirectly working on the core belief from the beginning of treatment. A belief of helplessness, for example, can be attenuated when patients set goals, modify their thematically-related automatic thoughts, successfully engage in mastery experiences, and give themselves credit. Beliefs of unlovability may start to shift when therapists help patients engage in rewarding social interactions and treat them in a warm, empathic, and caring manner.

Belief modification is more likely to be successful when patients believe (1) they can trust their therapist, (2) the process will help, and (3) the outcome of belief modification will lead to a better life. Otherwise patients may have a negative reaction when their therapist engages them in evaluating their core beliefs. The narcissistic patient, for example, may feel belittled, the borderline patient may feel too vulnerable, the histrionic patient may feel too unspecial. These patients may then use their usual coping strategies, becoming angry at the therapist, avoiding the topic, discussing beliefs superficially, or even skipping sessions or dropping out of treatment.

The first part of this chapter describes how to use and vary standard strategies to help patients modify their core beliefs about the self (see also Chapter 2). A final section focuses on helping patients modify core beliefs about other people. Helen, a patient introduced in the previous chapter, is also used as an example throughout this chapter.

USING AND VARYING STANDARD STRATEGIES TO MODIFY CORE BELIEFS

Therapists may need to use many strategies over a long period of time to help some patients with challenging problems alter their core beliefs. Among other techniques, therapists may use Socratic questioning, changing a comparison of the self, cognitive continua, acting "as if," developing role models, rational-emotional role plays, environmental interventions, family involvement, group therapy, dreams and metaphors, and imagery to restructure the meaning of traumatic childhood experiences. These techniques are described below.

Educating Patients about Core Beliefs and Coping Strategies

Therapists need to educate patients about core beliefs, incorporating important concepts such as the following:

- Core beliefs, like automatic thoughts and assumptions, are ideas, not truths.
- Patients may believe their core beliefs so thoroughly that they phrase these ideas almost as emotions ("I *feel* totally incompetent"; "I *feel* inferior"; "I *feel* unlovable").
- Patients develop certain behaviors to cope with these beliefs, behaviors that lead them to act in dysfunctional ways in some situations.
- Given patients' adverse childhood experiences, it is understandable why they would develop such extreme dysfunctional beliefs and coping strategies. Their beliefs may or may not have been completely valid during childhood. Regardless of their historical validity, they may certainly be largely or nearly completely invalid today.
- Patients can evaluate the validity of their core beliefs, and, if they find them to be distorted, can modify them to reflect reality more closely.
- The process of modifying core beliefs will likely be anxiety-provoking in the short run. Ultimately patients will feel better about themselves and be better able to achieve their goals.

Linking Core Beliefs with Coping Strategies

Before they are ready to start evaluating and modifying their core beliefs, many patients can benefit from their therapist's drawing a diagram that explains how the core belief affects their behavior and how these coping strategies in turn reinforce the core belief.

THERAPIST: (*drawing*) Does this seem right, Helen? You have a belief that you are defective, which you accept as true, without thinking to question it, and as a result, you avoid doing a lot of things that you think you'll fail at, and avoiding these things makes you feel more defective, which makes you avoid more. (*pause*) Did I get that right?

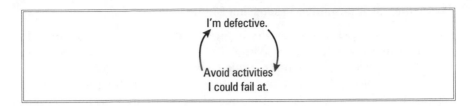

I'm defective.

Avoid activities
I could fail at.

If patients confirm the pattern, therapists can demonstrate how this pattern lays the groundwork for their perceptions and behavior in everyday situations. When therapists judge that patients are ready, they can bring a blank conceptualization diagram (see Chapter 2) into the session to be filled out with the patient—or the therapist can elaborate the diagram above, as follows:

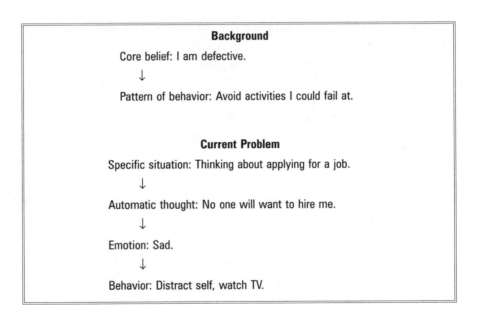

Background

Core belief: I am defective.

↓

Pattern of behavior: Avoid activities I could fail at.

Current Problem

Specific situation: Thinking about applying for a job.

↓

Automatic thought: No one will want to hire me.

↓

Emotion: Sad.

↓

Behavior: Distract self, watch TV.

Posing a Therapeutic Hypothesis

Therapists can then pose a dichotomous therapeutic hypothesis about the patient's core belief:

THERAPIST: Either the problem is that you really *are* completely [defective] and we'll have to work together to make you okay *OR* that's not the problem at all—the problem is that you have a *belief* that you are completely [defective]. We'll have to figure out together which is probably more accurate.

Presenting an Information-Processing Model

An information-processing model is often very helpful in explaining to patients why they believe their core beliefs so strongly—but why the core beliefs may not be true, or not completely true, as illustrated in the transcript below. Note that the circular figure with the rectangular opening represents the patient's *schema*, the mental structure that organizes information. The content of the schema is the patient's core belief.

THERAPIST: Is it okay if we talk a little bit more about this idea you have that you're defective?

HELEN: Okay.

THERAPIST: You know, we've talked before about how this idea comes up day after day for you. Right?

HELEN: Right.

THERAPIST: And how you've believed it for a very long time.

HELEN: Yeah.

THERAPIST: I have a theory about why you believe it so strongly. (*pause*) But you have to tell me whether you think I'm right or wrong. Okay?

HELEN: Yeah.

THERAPIST: (*drawing diagram below*) Okay. Helen, it's almost as if there's a part of your mind that's shaped like this—you see it's like a circle with a rectangular opening.

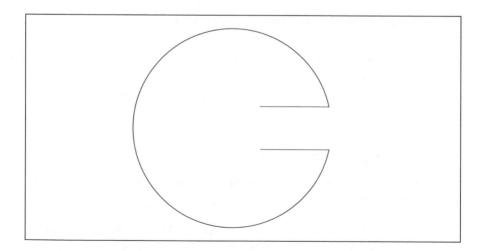

THERAPIST: (*writing*) And inside this part of your mind is the idea, "I am defective."

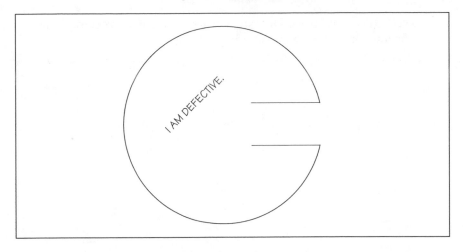

THERAPIST: Now let's say something happens. Let's see, you told me before that you went to church but you didn't talk to anyone. When you realized that you weren't talking, what did you say to yourself? Did you say, "What does this mean? Does it mean I'm defective? Does it mean I'm okay? Is it irrelevant?"

HELEN: I felt really abnormal.

THERAPIST: Did you have to think about it?

HELEN: No, I immediately felt like that.

THERAPIST: (*drawing*) So it's as if this event—not talking to anyone at church—is contained in a negative rectangle.

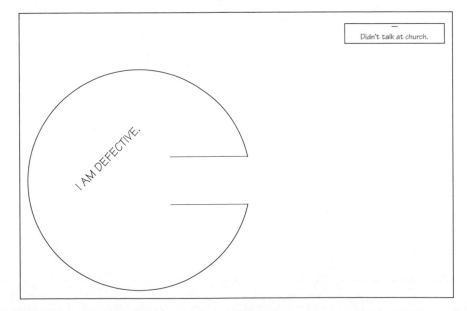

THERAPIST: (*drawing arrow*) Do you see how since it's a rectangle, it fits right into the rectangular opening?

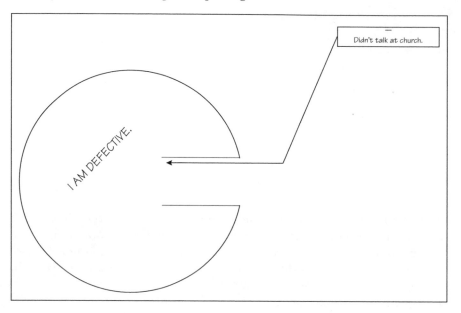

THERAPIST: (*underlining "I am defective"*) And every time a rectangle goes in, it makes this idea "I am defective" stronger.

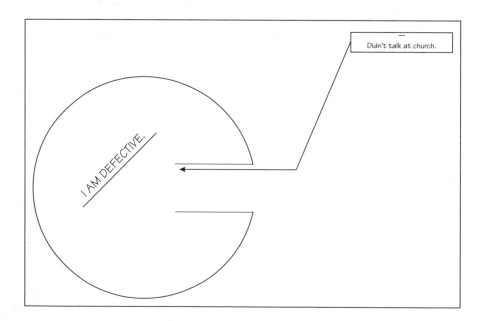

HELEN: Yeah.

THERAPIST: Let's try another situation . . . . Let's see. You said last week that you hadn't balanced your checkbook and you got overdrawn at the bank. When that happened, did you say to yourself, "That means I'm defective—or that means I'm okay—or getting overdrawn isn't relevant to that?

HELEN: No, I immediately thought, "What an idiot. I'm hopeless."

THERAPIST: (*drawing and underlining*) So getting overdrawn is also a negative rectangle and it goes right in . . . and makes the idea "I am defective" stronger.

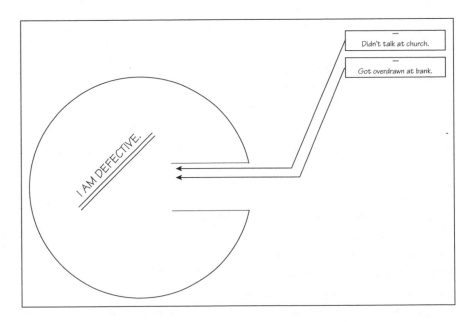

THERAPIST: Let's try one more. When else this week did you feel defective?

HELEN: (*Thinks.*) Sunday night. I stayed in all day Sunday even though the weather was beautiful.

THERAPIST: And when you realized you had spent the entire day inside, what did that mean to you?

HELEN: That there was really something wrong with me.

THERAPIST: So it looks like the defectiveness belief had kicked in again.

HELEN: Yeah.

THERAPIST: (*drawing and underlying*) So that follows the same pattern . . . .

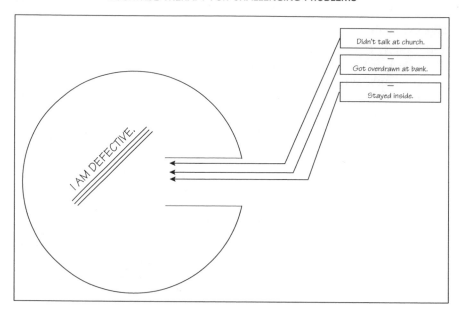

THERAPIST: Okay, so what do you think of this theory? Whenever anything happens or you do anything that could possibly mean that
you're defective, that information immediately goes straight to this
part of your mind (*pointing to diagram*), without your even thinking
much about it. (*pause*) Do you think that could be right?

HELEN: Yeah, I can see that.

THERAPIST: You're not just saying that?

HELEN: No, no. I think that's right.

THERAPIST: Okay. Here's my second theory. When anything happens or
you do anything that could possibly mean you're *okay*, that information
doesn't go straight in. I think something else happens to it. (*pause*) For
example, you told me a few minutes ago that your friend Jean wanted
you to help her pick out presents for her family because she thinks you
have good taste. (*pause*) When she asked you, did you say to yourself,
"Oh, good, if she wants my help, she must think I'm okay?"

HELEN: No.

THERAPIST: What did you say?

HELEN: That she must be hard up if she wants *me* to go.

THERAPIST: (*drawing*) So here something *good* happened—but it's as if this
information is in a triangle.

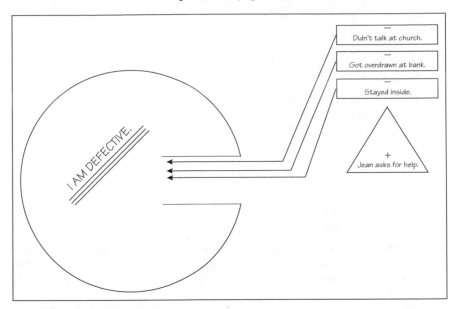

THERAPIST: Do you see, the triangle can't fit in the rectangular opening? It has to get *changed* to get in. So you said to yourself, "She must be hard up if she wants me to go," and the positive triangle changed to a negative rectangle. (*drawing*) Now it can fit in . . . . Do you see that?

HELEN: Yeah.

THERAPIST: (*underlines "I am defective" again*) And it strengthens the defective idea more.

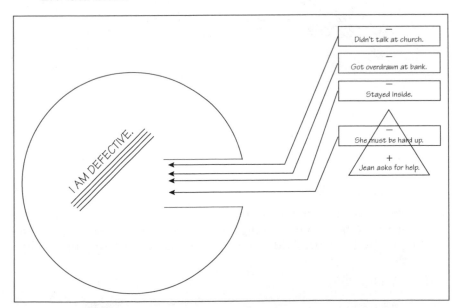

HELEN: Yeah.

THERAPIST: Let's see if we can come up with any other examples. What did you do this week that *I* would say showed you were okay, not defective.

HELEN: (*Thinks.*) I did start learning to do some word processing on Jean's computer.

THERAPIST: That's great! And did you say to yourself, "That's really good. Here I am, learning this stuff on the computer?

HELEN: No, nothing like that.

THERAPIST: What did you say to yourself?

HELEN: That it's pitiful. I'm probably the only one I know who doesn't already know how to do it.

THERAPIST: (*drawing as he speaks*) Oh, sounds like the same thing happened. Here you had a positive event, a positive triangle, and it had to get changed into a negative rectangle to fit in. Is that right?

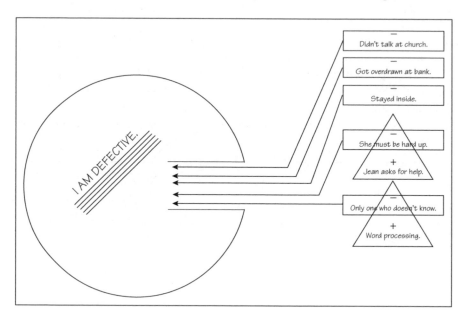

HELEN: Yeah. I guess so.

THERAPIST: Let's take one more example. (*pause*) Let's see. You told me that you've been getting things done around your apartment, painting the walls, getting rid of old clothes and stuff, fixing the kitchen table.

HELEN: Yeah.

THERAPIST: And when you did that stuff, did you immediately think, "That shows I'm okay—not defective"?

HELEN: (*Thinks.*) No, I don't think I thought anything of it.

THERAPIST: But if you *hadn't* done those things, then would you have thought you were defective?

HELEN: Yeah, probably.

THERAPIST: (*drawing*) So here are some positive triangles that just bounce off. You didn't really realize that these things were positive.

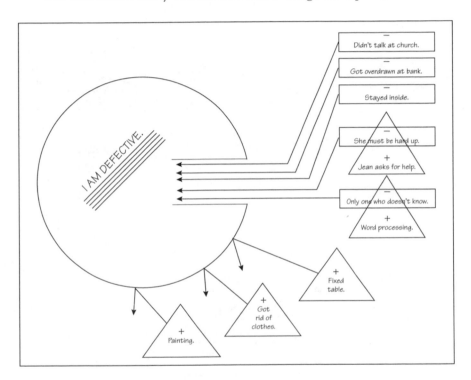

THERAPIST: What do you think of this theory? That almost anything you do, or anything that happens to you that is positive, either gets changed into a negative or it bounces off; you just don't notice it.

HELEN: (*Thinks.*) Yeah . . . I guess. . . that seems about right.

THERAPIST: And so what happens over time? If you keep seeing things over and over again as negative—and either don't notice positives or change them into negatives—do you see how this idea that you're defective could get stronger and stronger and stronger—and yet might not be true?

HELEN: (*Thinks.*) I don't know . . . . It makes sense.

THERAPIST: Well, it's something to think about. (*pause*) What do you think about, for homework, if you try to notice these kinds of positive and negative events and see what happens, how you interpret them? Would that be all right?

HELEN: Yeah.

THERAPIST: (*drawing*) Here, you could write them right on this sheet. Put the negative events that immediately make you feel like you're defective in the left column under the rectangle. And put the positive events in the right column under the triangle.

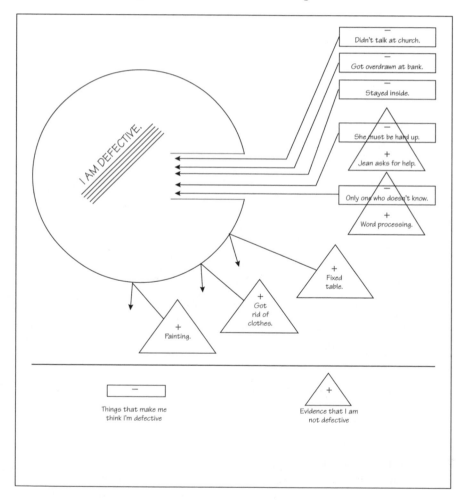

THERAPIST: Next week we can talk about how you can learn to interrupt this pattern. Does that sound okay?

At the end of the session, the therapist asked Helen to summarize
what she had learned and write it on a card:

> The idea that I am defective gets stronger and stronger
> because everyday I take situations to mean that I'm an idiot,
> or abnormal, or that there's something wrong with me. And I
> ignore or discount positive events that show the opposite.
> Each time I do that, it strengthens the idea that I'm
> defective. I can learn how to undo this in therapy.

The basic diagram can be supplemented by a positive schema drawing. For example, if the patient already incorporates some positive data
contrary to the core belief, the therapist can draw a smaller diagram
below the one that contains the negative core belief, provide it with a tri-
angular opening, and label it with the adaptive belief.

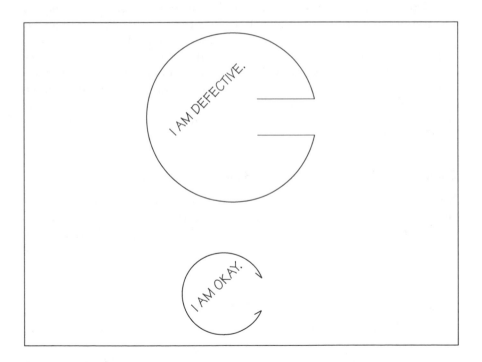

Or if the patient processes data positively, but it does not seem to "stick," the therapist can draw the second diagram with a trapdoor.

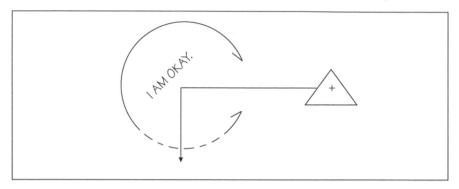

Using Analogies

Analogies can also help get across the idea that core beliefs are merely very strong ideas. Helen's therapist used an example of the people before Columbus's time who so firmly believed that the world was flat that they never tested the idea and made sure to avoid sailing too far from land. Helen's therapist also questioned her about people who held a prejudice that she did not share. She was able to see how a neighbor with extremely conservative views fixed on data that supported her ideas and discounted or ignored ideas to the contrary. Helen was able to see that her own belief of defectiveness was actually a strong prejudice against herself (see Padesky, 1993).

Constructing More Realistic Core Beliefs

It is desirable, at least initially, to help patients develop a new core belief that is not the opposite of the old core belief. Helen was able eventually to believe that she was "okay" much of the time. Another patient, Hal, adopted the belief that he was normal, with strengths and weaknesses like everyone else.

Motivating Patients to Change Core Beliefs

Therapists can increase patients' motivation to do the hard work of changing their core beliefs by helping them identify and record the advantages and disadvantages of changing their core beliefs. Additional important information may also be obtained by identifying advantages and disadvantages of *maintaining* the current core belief. During homework and therapy sessions, Helen continued to add to her lists in Figure 13.1. Her therapist helped her reframe her dysfunctional ideas.

Advantages of changing my core belief	Disadvantages of changing the core belief
• Feel better about myself. • Move ahead in life. • Get a boyfriend. • Get a job. • Have regular income. • Be able to buy things I want (a computer, a TV, CDs, clothes, etc.). • Be able to eat out more. • Won't feel inferior around my family. • Won't have to make excuses for not doing much. • Won't feel so anxious around other people. • Will want to do things other than watch TV. • Will be able to enjoy things more.	• I'll feel anxious BUT the anxiety will be time-limited. • I feel like I won't know who I am BUT it doesn't mean changing any good ideas I have about myself—only the "I am defective" idea. • I'll have to take risks BUT the rewards could be substantial. • I'll have to do hard things BUT my therapist will help me.
Advantages of maintaining my core belief (with reframes)	**Disadvantages of maintaining the core belief**
• I can avoid anxiety BUT I get anxious anyway and avoiding things makes me feel depressed and hopeless. • I don't have to take on challenges and maybe fail BUT I will continue to lead a boring, poor life, and, besides, therapy can help make the challenges easier. • It gives me a reason to stay home and watch television BUT watching TV is only a temporary distraction and I usually feel worse at the end of the day, when I realize how little I've gotten done. • Won't have to work hard in therapy BUT the potential payoff is great.	• Keeps me depressed. • Keeps me isolated from others. • Keeps me away from experiences that I could find satisfying. • Keeps me away from pleasurable activities. • Keeps me feeling guilty. • Keeps me feeling like a failure. • Keeps me from reaching my goals. • Keeps me from earning a regular paycheck. • Keeps me wasting my time and my life.

FIGURE 13.1. Advantages and disadvantages of changing and maintaining core beliefs.

Patients may also benefit from envisioning their life 10 years from now in detail, first when they have not changed their core belief, and so are 10 years older, more worn down, their lives even more impoverished or painful. Then therapists can help patients imagine their lives 10 years from now when they've had nearly 10 years of feeling good about themselves, acting functionally, with improved relationships and satisfying work and activities.

CASE EXAMPLE WITH BELIEF MODIFICATION TECHNIQUES

Many different kinds of techniques, described in *Cognitive Therapy: Basics and Beyond* (J. Beck,1995) and in the previous two chapters, are required to help patients modify their core beliefs over time. As in the previous section and chapter, Helen, a chronically depressed, formerly alcohol-dependent, unemployed woman, is used to illustrate major interventions in helping patients modify their core beliefs.

Recognizing the Activation of Core Beliefs

First, it was important for Helen to recognize when her core belief had been activated. Once her therapist introduced the idea of negatively perceived situations consonant with the core belief as a "negative rectangle," her therapist continually referred to them in this way. He asked her to pull out the following coping card they had jointly composed when she felt distressed or found herself trying to avoid becoming distressed:

> Am I believing again that I'm defective?
>
> If so, I've probably just experienced a negative rectangle. What is an alternative explanation or another view of the situation?

Her therapist also monitored the strength of Helen's core belief toward the beginning of therapy sessions and helped Helen identify "negative rectangles" that had arisen during the week that they should discuss during their session. He also became more conversational during the bridge, trying to identify positive triangles that Helen might not otherwise have spontaneously reported.

THERAPIST: Tell me more about your week. What were some good things that happened? What did you do? Anything pleasurable? Anything you felt good about? Did you spend any time with Jean or your sister?

Whenever they discussed a relevant problem during the session, the therapist tried to ascertain whether Helen's core belief had led to either undue distress or dysfunctional behavior:

THERAPIST: (*summarizing*) So your sister's friend called you about a possible job, but you didn't call him back. Do you think your core belief of defectiveness got in the way?

Changing the Processing of Negative Information

After Helen had confirmed that the model seemed to represent how she processed information, her therapist started to teach her how to respond to each piece of negative data, by writing the word "BUT" next to each rectangle. He then Socratically questioned her to help her formulate a plausible alternative explanation or an alternate way of viewing the event. For example:

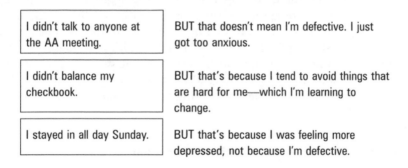

I didn't talk to anyone at the AA meeting.	BUT that doesn't mean I'm defective. I just got too anxious.
I didn't balance my checkbook.	BUT that's because I tend to avoid things that are hard for me—which I'm learning to change.
I stayed in all day Sunday.	BUT that's because I was feeling more depressed, not because I'm defective.

Helen's therapist helped her see that the "negative rectangles" were really the "situation" part of the cognitive model and that looking for alternative explanations or viewpoints was similar to the second question on the Dysfunctional Thought Record. He had her keep a running list of negative rectangle data, with a response for each item that reflected the core belief.

Helen's therapist suggested a technique to help Helen reframe these negative rectangles at home. If she could not think of an alternative viewpoint, she could ask herself:

"What would [Jean/my sister/my therapist] say about this?"

Her therapist also helped her see that her interpretation of herself as defective in many situations stemmed from what Helen imagined her *father* would have said to her. Perceiving her automatic response as coming from a highly critical and unreliable source helped reduce its validity in her mind.

In order to help Helen counter some of her negative rectangles, her therapist provided her with additional psychoeducation. One difficulty Helen had was making herself do everyday things, such as getting up early, keeping her apartment clean, paying her bills on time—in essence, disciplining herself to do things she did not want to do. She had always seen her difficulties as meaning that she was lazy and defective.

Through psychoeducation, her therapist helped her understand how it is that children learn to internalize self-discipline and tolerate frustration through the structures their parents provide. She came to understand that reasonable parents monitor what their children do (e.g., completing their homework), reinforce them for being productive, and impose reasonable consequences when their children fail to fulfill their responsibilities. They help their children structure their time and give them tasks to do to help the family function well. Over time, these parents give children increasing responsibilities at home. Children learn to do things they do not want to do; they learn not to struggle with their parents or themselves about doing the essentials—in essence, they learn not to give themselves *choices* about whether or not to do certain things. These structures were almost completely absent in Helen's childhood household. Her therapist helped her see that it was no wonder that she had difficulty disciplining herself as an adult. He helped her reframe her idea that she was lazy and defective; rather, she was lacking in some specific skills that she could learn.

Changing the Processing of Positive Information

It was also important for Helen to recognize when she was discounting or ignoring positive data. Her therapist helped her change the form of the discount. For example, one of Helen's positive triangles that had changed into a negative rectangle contained the idea:

"I helped Jean put up bookshelves but anyone could do that."

Her therapist helped her discount her discount:

"BUT Jean couldn't do it. It's evidence I'm *not* defective."

Her therapist had her write this adaptive response in her running list of "positive triangle" items. Other examples included:

"I went to a job interview but I probably won't get it," BUT it's good that I went in any case.

"I cleaned up part of my apartment but I didn't do it very well," BUT I succeeded in doing some of it.

It was difficult for Helen to recognize positive data that she took for granted. As time went on, and she behaved more and more functionally, Helen actually had a lot of data to support her new core belief that she was okay. She also *refrained* from doing many dysfunctional things. Helen's therapist asked the following questions, then had her write her responses in new triangles for her list:

■ "Can you imagine that I followed you around this week? What did you do that I would notice and say, 'Hey, that goes to show that you're okay'?"
■ "What did you do this week that if [your friend/family member/roommate/coworker/neighbor] had done it, you could have pointed to it and said, 'This shows he or she is okay'?"

Examining Information Processing Historically

Helen's therapist also helped her realize that she had been screening *in* negative data and screening *out* or discounting positive data ever since she was a child. He asked her to recall negative and positive data from specific childhood periods—elementary school, pre-school, high school, and beyond. He had her record this data on a running "historical negative rectangle" list and a "historic positive triangle" list for each period.

Both in session, and for homework, Helen reframed the historical negative data and the discounted positive data. Her therapist also had her look at photographs and interview a caring aunt and uncle with whom she had spent some time as a child. Doing so helped her identify new "positive triangles." Her therapist and she then reviewed the accumulated data from each period and drew adaptive conclusions.

Through this process, Helen was able to grasp, for example, that her poor performance toward the end of elementary school did not mean she was defective. Through Socratic questioning, she concluded that it was more likely related to the emotional upheaval she was experiencing at home—given her father's alcoholism and physical abuse and her mother's depressed withdrawal. She was able to see that giving up was a natural response to an extremely stressful environment.

Socratic Questioning

Along with questions designed to reframe the "negative rectangles" (and the discounting of "positive triangles") and to identify other "positive triangles," Helen's therapist continually asked her questions to evaluate her core belief generally and in the context of specific problems. A few—of the *multitude* of questions he asked in the course of therapy—are listed below.

General Questions

- "What does 'defective' mean?"
- "Here's *my* definition of defective . . . .What do you think about that?"
- "If someone has a history of depression, does that necessarily mean she is *defective*—couldn't it mean she has an illness?"
- "If it turned out that your nephew grew up in traumatic circumstances and became depressed for many years, would you want *him* to view himself as defective? How would you *want* him to see himself?"
- (*after reviewing Helen's childhood experiences*) "Well, no *wonder* you grew up believing you were defective. Wouldn't you think almost any kid in these circumstances would believe that about herself? Can you see that even though she might believe it very strongly, it might not be true?
- "Isn't it possible that people can have weaknesses, even a lot of weaknesses, without being defective as human beings?"

Questions about the Use of Dysfunctional Coping Strategies

- "Do you think your belief that you are defective got activated [in this situation]?"
- "Do you think you could have [behaved in this dysfunctional way] because you *felt* defective?"
- "Is this [dysfunctional behavior] another negative rectangle?"
- "How can you respond now to this rectangle?"
- "If you had not felt defective, do you think you might have done something different? What would that have been?"
- "What would a *truly* defective person have done in this situation?"

Questions about Using More Functional Behavior

- "What do you make of the fact that you [displayed adaptive behavior in this situation instead of your usual coping strategy]?"
- "Is it possible you're not as defective as you feel?"

Therapy Notes

At nearly every session, Helen's therapist helped her draw conclusions that she wrote on index cards. Throughout their sessions, her therapist continually asked himself:

■ "What does Helen need to remember this week?"

Reviewing these cards everyday at home was an important part of Helen's effort to integrate her new, more functional ideas.

Changing the Comparison

Helen continually became demoralized when she compared herself to her sister, her high school classmates, her friend Jean, and her neighbors. Her therapist helped her recognize the negative impact of these comparisons on her mood, her motivation, and her behavior. They decided that when she caught herself making this kind of comparison, she should immediately change it. She could compare herself instead to how she had been during a particularly low period in her life—and recall how different she was now and how much progress she had made in her life since that point.

Cognitive Continuum

When Helen arrived at a particular therapy session, she was quite upset. She had just come from her parents' house where her father had belittled her in the presence of her sister and nephew for having only a part-time, low-skilled job, not being married, and being childless. When her therapist asked how defective she felt, Helen replied 100%. Her therapist began to draw a scale. (See Figure 13.2 for the final version of the scale.)

THERAPIST: So you feel 100% defective. Could there be anyone who is more defective than you?

HELEN: (*with her head in her hands*) I don't know. I don't know.

THERAPIST: (*Waits.*)

HELEN: (*finally*) Yeah, I guess. We've talked about him before: Fred.

THERAPIST: (*emphasizing the features Helen found particularly undesirable*) The guy you know who beats his wife, beats his kids, and is on disability even though his back is now fine?

HELEN: Yeah.

THERAPIST: So if he's 100% defective, where does that put you?

HELEN: 90%, I guess.

THERAPIST: (*Crosses off Helen's name on the scale, replaces it with "Fred," and writes Helen's name further down the scale.*) Anybody more defective than Fred?

HELEN: A murderer, I guess.

THERAPIST: (*proposing a specific person*) Like the guy, Joe something, I think his name is, the one here in this neighborhood with a little kid who killed his wife for the insurance money?

HELEN: Yeah, him.

THERAPIST: So, where would you put Joe?

HELEN: Well, he'd have to be 100%.

THERAPIST: So where would that put Fred?

HELEN: (*Thinks.*) Down more. Maybe 70%.

THERAPIST: And you—where do you go on this scale?

HELEN: 50%, I guess.

THERAPIST: (*Continues to cross out prior items on the scale and positions them according to Helen's new designations.*) And where in terms of defectiveness would you put someone like Saddam Hussein?

HELEN: Oh, he's definitely at 100%.

THERAPIST: Then where does this move Joe the murderer?

HELEN: 90%, I guess.

THERAPIST: Who's between Joe the murderer and Fred?

HELEN: Ummm. A rapist, I guess.

THERAPIST: And between a rapist and Fred?

HELEN: I don't know. A child molester.

THERAPIST: So where would the rapist and the child molester be? Where would Fred be? Where would you be?

HELEN: (*Moves everyone down; she now puts herself at 40%.*)

THERAPIST: And who might be between you and Fred?

HELEN: (*Thinks.*) I'm not sure.

THERAPIST: How about someone who's not quite as defective as Fred, but someone who is clearly not okay? Like an unemployed person, without depression or any other kind of problem, who has a family but is really selfish, just doesn't want to work and his family is living in poverty?

HELEN: Yeah, that's bad.

THERAPIST: Where would he go?

HELEN: Ummm, maybe 40%.

THERAPIST: And I'm just curious. Where would you put your father?

HELEN: (*Looks at scale.*) He'd be 40%, too.

THERAPIST: Even though he's working, and is married, and has a family?

HELEN: Yeah. Yeah. He's defective in other ways.

THERAPIST: And where are you on the scale now?

HELEN: About 20%, I guess.

THERAPIST: And where do you think *I'd* put you on the scale?

HELEN: Well, you've said before you don't think I'm defective.

THERAPIST: So I'd put you at zero.

HELEN: Yeah.

THERAPIST: Right. Let's put that in, too. (*Writes it down.*) Helen, how are you feeling now?

HELEN: Better.

THERAPIST: So what idea changed?

HELEN: (*Takes a deep breath.*) I guess my father was making me feel really defective. But maybe I'm not. Maybe he's more defective than me. (*pause*) Maybe there *are* other people who are more defective than me.

THERAPIST: I wonder if for homework you could think of anyone else who belongs on this scale.

HELEN: (*Nods.*)

THERAPIST: And could you think about something we've talked about be-

---

Defectiveness Scale

100%—Saddam Hussein
 90%—Joe (murderer)
 80%—rapist
 70%—child molester
 60%—wife batterer
 50%—big time drug dealer
 40%—Fred, dad
 30%—corrupt official
 20%—Helen (according to herself)
 10%—hypocritical preacher
  0%—Helen (according to therapist)

FIGURE 13.2. Cognitive continuum.

fore: that maybe you don't really belong on a "Defective Scale"?
Maybe you belong on a scale for people who really are okay but suffer
from depression.

HELEN: Yeah.

Acting "As If"

When Helen reported that she had to go to a family wedding, her therapist used the opportunity to have her envision what she would do if she
did not believe that her old core belief, but rather believed her new, more
adaptive belief.

THERAPIST: So, Helen, if you truly believed that you were not defective, in
    fact that you were truly okay, what would you do at your cousin's wed-
    ding reception this weekend? . . . Would you get there on time? . . .
    How would you look as you went in the ballroom? . . . What would
    your posture be like? . . . How would your face look? . . . What would
    you do when you saw your cousin? . . . His bride? . . . What would you
    say to her family? . . . What would you say to your relatives? . . . To the
    friends of your family? . . . What would you say to someone you didn't
    know?

Following this discussion, Helen's therapist rehearsed with her what she
could say to herself before and during the event to make it more likely that
she could engage in these more functional behaviors.

Developing a Role Model

Helen's therapist asked her to think of a positive role model to emulate—
both in terms of thinking and behaving—in certain situations. He suggested that her role model might be someone she knew, a character in a
movie or in literature, or a public figure. They decided it would be helpful to think about how Helen' friend Jean would view herself in certain
situations—for example, when she made a mistake or had to go to a social
gathering where she did not know anyone. "If Jean had overdrawn her
account, what would she have said?" "If Jean were going to the church
social, where she didn't know anyone, what would she do?"

Rational-Emotional Role Plays

After considerable work on attenuating her old core belief and reinforcing her new one, Helen revealed that she could see intellectually to a large
degree that she was not defective, but still felt emotionally (or in her gut)

that she was defective. Her therapist did a rational-emotional role play (see J. Beck, 1995, for a full description).

THERAPIST: How much do you still believe you're defective?

HELEN: Not that much—intellectually. I don't know. In my gut, it still feels like I am.

THERAPIST: Can we do a role play? I'd like to play the part of your mind that knows you're not defective and I'd like you to play the emotional part that still feels defective, and I'd like you to argue against me as strongly as you can, to convince me that you are defective. Would that be okay?

HELEN: Yeah.

THERAPIST: Okay, you start. Say, "I'm defective because . . . " and I'll answer you back.

HELEN: (*Sighs.*) I'm defective. I have this lousy, low-paying job, and I'm not married, don't have a family . . . I'm nothing.

THERAPIST: That's not true. I'm not nothing. I'm a normal person. I don't have a lot of things that I really want because my depression held me back for a lot of years, but that doesn't mean I'm defective.

HELEN: Just having depression makes me defective.

THERAPIST: No, it doesn't. No more than having a medical condition like a bad heart makes someone defective. It's true that I've missed out on some important life experiences but it doesn't say anything about me as a person.

HELEN: (*silent*)

THERAPIST: (*out of role play*) Now argue back against me. Convince me I'm wrong, that you are defective.

HELEN: But there must be something terribly wrong with me that I got depressed and stayed depressed and wasted so many years.

THERAPIST: There has been something wrong with me. I've been depressed!

HELEN: But some depressed people get married and have families and hold down jobs and don't become alcoholic like I did.

THERAPIST: That's true. They had different genes and were born with a different personality and had different life experiences. Some depressed people cope better than I do and some cope worse—but it doesn't mean that the higher functioning ones are okay and I'm defective.

HELEN: (*silent*)

THERAPIST: (*out of role play*) Keep arguing.

HELEN: But I don't have a life. Normal people have lives.

THERAPIST: It's true that I don't have the life that I want—yet. But I do have a life—and I'm making it better all the time. In the last few months, I got a job, I'm doing the job, I moved, I've started to meet people at church, I'm getting stuff done around the house.

HELEN: But I should have done all these things years ago.

THERAPIST: I wish I could have. And if I had had different treatment for my depression years ago, maybe I could have. It's unfortunate I didn't.

HELEN: (*silent*)

THERAPIST: Can you keep arguing?

HELEN: (*Thinks.*) I can't think of anything else.

THERAPIST: Okay. Can we switch parts now? I'd like you to be the intellectual part that knows that you're really okay and I'll be the emotional part that still feels defective.

HELEN: Okay.

THERAPIST: I'll start . . . I know I'm defective. I have this lousy job, it doesn't pay very well. I'm not married, don't have any kids . . . I'm nothing.

They continued the role play until Helen's therapist had repeated all the emotional arguments that Helen had used in the first part of the role play. At times he had to exaggerate the emotional arguments or break out of the role play to discuss an adaptive response when Helen got stuck. A few sessions later, he used a variation of this technique, in which he asked Helen to play both parts of her mind:

THERAPIST: (*summarizing*) So when you opened your paycheck and saw how much it was for, you thought, "I really am a loser," which meant to you that you were defective?

HELEN: Yeah.

THERAPIST: What does your head say to that?

HELEN: That I'm doing better. At least I have a full-time job now.

THERAPIST: And what does your gut say to that?

HELEN: That it's still only minimum wage.

THERAPIST: And what does your head say to that?

HELEN: What we talked about, I guess. That it's a stepping-stone to something better. That a few months ago I was spending most of my days in bed.

THERAPIST: What does your gut say about that?

HELEN: That it's pathetic to have to start at the bottom.

THERAPIST: And what does your head say to that?

HELEN: (*Thinks.*) I guess . . . that it's not pathetic. When you've been depressed for as long as I've been, it's pretty good.

THERAPIST: And what does your gut say to that?

HELEN: (*Thinks.*) Nothing, I guess. It's quiet.

THERAPIST: Good!

Environmental Changes

As therapy progressed and her depression lifted somewhat, Helen became increasingly demoralized by her apartment. It was small, dark, and cramped and was located in a deteriorating neighborhood. With much trepidation, but with support from her therapist and her friend, Jean, Helen investigated other living situations. It became apparent that she would need to share living quarters if she wanted to move to a better section of the city. She eventually found a house near a university; two graduate students who were already living in a house were looking for an additional housemate. Although the physical move and the initial adjustment were difficult, it turned out to be a good decision. Helen got along especially well with one housemate and was a little irritated by the second. But Helen's daily routines, social life, and involvement in activities increased significantly. She had to abide by the house rules, so she could not procrastinate about doing dishes, cleaning the bathroom, and straightening up common areas. Her housemates sometimes invited her along when they attended events. She had someone to talk to in the evening. Helen slowly began to feel more and more normal.

Family Involvement

After carefully assessing the benefits and risks, Helen and her therapist decided to invite her sister, Julie, to part of a session, to get her perspective on Helen. After providing some psychoeducation and reviewing how Helen's depression had affected Helen, the therapist gently questioned Julie. In response, Julie said how sorry she was that depression had taken such a toll on Helen. She noted several positive changes in her in the previous few months. She expressed anger toward their father, how he had treated Helen as a child and continued to treat her now. Julie stated that she did not see Helen as defective, but as someone who had struggled for a long time. She asked how she could be more helpful to Helen. Helen was quite moved and was able to process and believe much of what her sister said. Following this session, Julie and Helen talked more regularly by phone and saw one another once or twice a month. Julie's continued expressions of support and caring constituted important "positive triangles."

Group Therapy

Although Helen did not elect to engage in group therapy or get involved with a support group, these kinds of experiences are often very helpful in providing patients with reframes for their negative rectangles and with data for positive triangles, as they start to see that other people with difficulties are not defective, or bad, or unlovable, or helpless. Perceiving that other people struggle and that other people can overcome their difficulties can help patients gain hope and a new perspective on themselves.

Dreams and Metaphors

About 6 weeks after the start of therapy, Helen reported a dream that she had had the previous night. She was dressed in rags, standing by the side of a fast-flowing river, desperately wanting to cross, but being afraid she would drown. The therapist probed for Helen's associations and meanings. Helen expressed a theme of helplessness, of wanting to improve her life, but being too frightened to try. Her rags seemed to represent a theme of defectiveness. She agreed to discuss the dream at greater length, to look for a way to improve it. Helen liked her therapist's suggestion of imagining building a bridge across the river, which represented reaching her goals.

They decided that the first step would be to envision what the bridge would look like. Helen initially described a very high and elaborate span. After some discussion, she decided that a low bridge would suffice, be easier to build, and be less scary to cross.

Helen said that she would first need to build two stone supports resting on the bottom of the river, one toward the closer riverbank and the other closer to the opposite side. She and her therapist decided that these supports were already partly in place and were visible slightly above the surface of the river. The stones were Helen's strengths, assets, and resources: her intelligence, her caring, her willingness to ask for help, her native persistence (e.g., in becoming and staying sober), her strong friendship with Jean, her improving relationship with her sister, her willingness to work in therapy, and the skills she had learned in therapy and in previous jobs.

They decided the next step would be for Helen to collect additional stones, put them in a rowboat, and row them to the first support. When Helen became worried that she would not have the strength to do that much work, her therapist asked whether she wanted to imagine getting help. She was visibly relieved when she realized she did not have to build the bridge alone. They talked about what the new stones represented and decided that they would be the new skills Helen would learn—especially how to consistently engage in adaptive, everyday behaviors (getting out of bed by 9 A.M., doing household chores, exercising, doing errands).

They also discussed what to do about the fast-flowing currents, deciding that these represented automatic thoughts that, untended, could slow down or even upset her boat: "I'll never get better. It [therapy] isn't going to work. What's the use? It's not worth trying. Things won't work out anyway." They discussed how if Helen gave credence to these thoughts, they would carry her down the river, further and further away from the bridge. She recognized that she would have to adaptively respond to her negative thinking, concentrate on both the big picture of the bridge, leading her where she wanted to go, and on the tasks she had to do just that day in the process of building the bridge.

Having imagined building up the supports, Helen felt at a loss about how to proceed. When her therapist asked what she had done before, when building the supports seemed beyond her, she recognized that she could again seek help. He also helped her see that she was not defective for not knowing what to do—how could she know? She had not had any prior experiences in building a bridge. They decided she could go on the Internet to get more information, she could call an engineering company, and she could rent the special equipment she would need. She imagined herself starting the beginning of the span, sitting in the cab of a steam shovel, with Jean, her therapist, and an engineer with blueprints on the bank, guiding her and cheering her on.

When her therapist asked what she was thinking and feeling as she sat in the cab of the steam shovel, she expressed anxiety that she would not have enough stamina to build the whole span. Her therapist helped her imagine that the slope of the span was actually quite gentle. She was also able to recognize that the harder part would be at the beginning, as she was still learning what to do and building uphill, but that it would become much easier as soon as she reached midspan, because the bridge would be going down. Still, they agreed that it would be important to build just a little of the span each day so that Helen would not become overwhelmed or too fatigued.

Helen's therapist asked Helen to draw herself building the bridge at home and to see what thoughts and feelings came up. At the next session, Helen added other important elements to the physical drawing. They discussed her fear that as she built the bridge higher, she could fall off, which meant to her that if she took on bigger challenges, she would fail and become very depressed. They decided she should draw four rowboats, spaced equidistantly, anchored and tethered by ropes to the supports and to structures on the riverbanks. In this way, if she were to fall, she could grab onto a rope and pull herself to a boat. Each rowboat had oars, a small motor, emergency supplies, and a cell phone. The rowboats represented access to her external resources: Jean, her sister, her therapist. She and her therapist next discussed putting up guard rails on the bridge to prevent her falling off. The guard rails were additional skills she was learning in therapy.

This metaphorical image was one that Helen's therapist and she returned to time after time in therapy. "Concentrating on the bridge" and "making progress on the bridge" became shorthand ways of reminding Helen to focus her efforts and recognize how far she had come.

Restructuring the Meaning of Traumatic Childhood Experiences

Using imagery to restructure the meaning of childhood experiences can help patients integrate on an emotional level what they have learned on an intellectual level. Helen's therapist used this technique with her several times toward the end of therapy, after she had significantly changed her dysfunctional assumptions and beliefs—especially intellectually. He took advantage of times when Helen entered the session quite distressed, with her core beliefs significantly activated. This kind of intervention can affect patients' emotional-level understanding but only if their affect is at a moderately high level and their beliefs are activated.

On one particular day, Helen came to session practically in tears. She had just begun a new job and a coworker had sharply criticized her for making a mistake and causing more work for him. Helen's therapist ascertained the core beliefs that had been activated. Then, instead of focusing on this incident, he asked Helen to focus on her distress and to recall specific events from her childhood in which she had also felt the same way.

Helen related an experience with her father (actually one that she had previously recalled as a "negative rectangle" during a historical review). She described an incident that had occurred when she was about 7 years old. One Saturday afternoon in the fall, Helen was playing in an organized soccer game. Her father, obviously drunk, showed up during the second half. He began cursing at Helen for missing a kick. Then he began arguing loudly with another parent. When Helen came off the field, her father humiliated her, called her names, and dragged her off to the parking lot where he beat her.

Helen's therapist next had her tell the story again, but this time imagining it in her mind's eye as if she were now 7 years old, and as if it were actually happening right now. Her therapist questioned the younger Helen, using language a 7-year-old could understand, to maintain a moderately high degree of distress, uncover important details, and identify key automatic thoughts, beliefs, and emotions. "Seven-year-old Helen, how are you feeling now? What are you thinking now? Why is this happening?"

The therapist had Helen continue the image until the beating was over, they had arrived home, and Helen had retreated to a safer place (her bed). The therapist continued to question "7-year-old Helen" to make sure he had elicited the most important cognitions. Then he asked 7-year-old Helen if it was okay with her if her adult self came into the bedroom to talk to her about what had happened. When Helen agreed, he suggested that she see her adult self enter her room. He asked her where she wanted her older self to be: standing by the bed? sitting with her on the bed? sitting with her arm around her? Next he facilitated an extended dialogue between the younger self and the adult self (the equivalent of a rational-emotional role play). He asked the younger Helen what she wanted to ask her adult self, then asked the adult self to respond in language appropriate for a 7-year-old.

With some guidance from her therapist, the adult Helen told her younger self that she was not bad, that there was nothing wrong with her, that in fact she was a wonderful girl. Her older self explained that it was her father who had done a bad thing and reminded her younger self that her father *often* did bad things when he drank too much beer. The older Helen told her younger self that the other kids and their parents at the game felt badly for Helen. They did not think that there was anything wrong with her. They only thought there was something wrong with her father.

Helen's therapist coached her younger self to tell her older self what she disagreed with or what she did not believe, so the older self would have an opportunity to respond. He measured the strength of her beliefs and intensity of her emotions (in language a 7-year-old could understand). When the younger self felt somewhat better and no longer believed the negative ideas about herself as strongly, he gave the younger self a chance to ask her adult self more questions before saying good-bye. Her younger self asked whether her father would continue to beat her.

Helen's therapist guided the older self in saying that she was very sorry, that yes, her father would continue to beat her, but that the younger Helen would grow older and that the beatings would stop, and that one day the younger Helen and the adult Helen would come to therapy to get help—and that the adult Helen knew this, because she was really her younger self grown up. Her younger self asked her adult self if she would come back and help her again, and adult Helen agreed. Helen imagined her 7-year-old self walking her older self outside and getting a hug good-bye.

Following this imagery exercise, Helen's therapist debriefed her about the experience, and they discussed her change of belief at an emotional level. Then they considered how Helen could make use of what she had learned in the coming week, to prepare for episodes in which her belief of defectiveness might again become activated and what she had just learned that could help her respond to it more effectively. They repeated this kind of therapeutic experience to restructure the meaning of several other key memories. It was this kind of intervention that finally helped Helen integrate on an emotional level what she had already grasped on an intellectual level.

Descriptions of using imagery to modify emotional level understanding can also be found in J. Beck (1995), Edwards (1990), Holmes & Hackmann (2004), Layden et al (1993), Smucker & Dancu (1999), and Young, Klosko, & Weishaar (2003).

Bibliotherapy

Helen was not willing to follow through with homework assignments that involved bibliotherapy but she probably would have benefited from psychoeducation about beliefs in *Prisoners of Belief* (McKay & Fanning, 1991), *Reinventing Your Life* (Young & Klosko, 1993), *Mind over Mood* (Greenberger & Padesky, 1995), or *Getting Your Life Back* (Wright & Basco, 2001).

MODIFYING CORE BELIEFS ABOUT OTHERS

The same techniques to help patients modify core beliefs about themselves are also used in helping them modify core beliefs about other people. Helen held a general core belief "Others will be critical of me." As with her other beliefs, Helen's therapist ascertained the breadth, frequency, and strength of the belief. He conceptualized how the belief impacted her beliefs about herself ("If people are critical of me, they are probably right, because I am defective") and her behavior ("If I don't take on challenges, I won't fail, and others won't have the opportunity to criticize me").

He helped her examine the validity of the belief through standard Socratic questioning both in general and in specific situations: What's the evidence this belief is true? What's the evidence it might not be true, or not completely true? He helped her decatastrophize the belief, generally and in specific situations: "If it's true that they are critical of you, what's the worst that could happen? How could you cope? What's the best that could happen? What's the most realistic outcome?" He reviewed with her the impact of this belief both in the short run and the long run. Following these discussions, he helped Helen write cards with adaptive responses.

A cognitive continuum helped Helen break up her black-and-white thinking. She was able to see that only a very few people in her life had been highly critical of her, and that most people were only mildly critical, neutral, or not at all critical.

The therapeutic relationship was also an important vehicle of change. Initially, Helen assumed that her therapist would be critical of her, especially for not completing her homework assignments. As he reacted in a problem-solving (but not critical) way, she began to realize that her fears about him were unfounded. His acceptance provided additional data contrary to her belief.

Helen's therapist helped her develop a new, more realistic and more functional belief, which she wrote on a card:

> Not everyone is critical, like my dad. In fact, the only other people like him were [two previous bosses and two teachers in high school]. Most people who really know me (like Jean, Sharona, Wayne, and [my therapist]) are *not* critical.

SUMMARY

Asking many patients with challenging problems to question their core beliefs can undermine their sense of self. Naturally, the process leads to patients feeling quite anxious. Therefore, therapists need to choose their timing well and motivate patients to engage and collaborate with them. Many strategies are required over time to help patients change their core beliefs. Maintenance is difficult; therefore therapists will need to continually help patients reiterate what they learned on both an intellectual and emotional level, and to enact the new beliefs at the behavioral level, so that affect changes in a deep and durable way.

APPENDIX A

■■■■■■■

Resources, Training, and Supervision in Cognitive Therapy

This book was designed to help therapists conceptualize difficulties in treating patients and modify treatment so they can help their patients more effectively. Therapists should also seek out additional resources to maximize their effectiveness with patients with challenging problems. Sometimes readings will suffice but often therapists (and their patients) benefit from hands-on training or supervision. This appendix describes two organizations with the mission of promoting therapist growth in cognitive therapy.

BECK INSTITUTE FOR COGNITIVE THERAPY AND RESEARCH

The Beck Institute (www.beckinstitute.org) is a non-profit psychotherapy center dedicated to training, clinical care, and research in cognitive therapy. Aaron T. Beck, MD, and I founded this organization in suburban Philadelphia in 1994. Since that time, hundreds of mental health professionals have been trained in cognitive therapy through the Visitors and Extramural Training Programs. Cognitive therapy training has been brought to thousands more through our outreach programs to universities, national and international professional associations, hospitals and hospital systems, community mental health systems, managed care organizations, and primary care physician and nursing groups, among others.

In addition to information about these training programs, a number of other important features can be found on the website:

- Continually updated *reading/reference lists* for mental health professionals.
- *Educational materials* (videos, DVDs, worksheet packets, books, patient brochures).
- Current and archived copies of *Cognitive Therapy Today*, the Beck Institute

newsletter, containing cutting-edge articles about various aspects of cognitive therapy, including clinical practice, theory, research, and training/supervision.
- A list of cognitive therapy-oriented *journals*.
- Abstracts of *outcome research* in cognitive therapy.
- Information about the adult and youth *Beck Scales*.
- *Links* to other cognitive therapy organizations.

In addition, the website offers several features for consumers:

- *Referral information.*
- A specialized cognitive therapy *reading list*.
- *Articles* from the popular press.
- A downloadable pamphlet, *Questions and Answers about Cognitive Therapy.*

For information contact:

Beck Institute for Cognitive Therapy and Research
P. O. Box 2673
Bala Cynwyd, PA 19004
Phone: 610-664-3020
Fax: 610-664-4437
E-mail: beckinst@gim.net
Website: www.beckinstitute.org

THE ACADEMY OF COGNITIVE THERAPY

The Academy of Cognitive Therapy (www.academyofct.org) is another non-profit organization that serves as a resource for both consumers and professionals. It was founded in 1999 by prominent clinicians, educators, and researchers in cognitive therapy. Aaron T. Beck is its honorary president. The Academy's website provides:

- Listings of *training and supervision programs* for mental health professionals.
- Descriptions of *graduate, postgraduate, and internship programs* in psychology, psychiatry, social work, and psychiatric nursing that emphasize cognitive therapy.
- *Workshops* in cognitive therapy.
- Information and materials for *cognitive therapy training*.
- Essential and recommended *reading lists*.
- *Therapist assessment tools* (such as the Cognitive Therapy Rating Scale and manual and the Cognitive Case Write-Up).
- Abstracts of selected *research articles*.
- Current and archived *newsletters* (*Advances in Cognitive Therapy*).
- *Links* to other cognitive therapy organizations.

This website also contains information pertinent to consumers, including:

- A worldwide *referral list* of certified cognitive therapists.
- *Fact sheets* on various psychiatric disorders.
- *Self-help materials.*
- *Reading lists.*

For information, contact:

Academy of Cognitive Therapy
Phone: 610-664-1273
Fax: 610-664-5137
E-mail: info@academyofct.org
Website: www.academyofct.org

APPENDIX B

Personality Belief Questionnaire

For information on the development, administration, and scoring of the Personality Belief Questionnaire, visit www.beckinstitute.org.

Name _____   Date: _____

Please read the statements below and rate HOW MUCH YOU BELIEVE EACH ONE. Try to judge how you feel about each statement MOST OF THE TIME.

4	3	2	1	0
I believe it totally	I believe it very much	I believe it moderately	I believe it slightly	I don't believe it at all

Example	How much do you believe it?				
1. The world is a dangerous place.	4 Totally	3 Very much	2 Mod- erately	1 Slightly	0 Not at all
1. I am socially inept and socially undesirable in work or social situations.	4	3	2	1	0
2. Other people are potentially critical, indifferent, demeaning, or rejecting.	4	3	2	1	0
3. I cannot tolerate unpleasant feelings.	4	3	2	1	0
4. If people get close to me, they will discover the "real" me and reject me.	4	3	2	1	0
5. Being exposed as inferior or inadequate will be intolerable.	4	3	2	1	0
6. I should avoid unpleasant situations at all cost.	4	3	2	1	0
7. If I feel or think something unpleasant, I should try to wipe it out or distract myself (for example, think of something else, have a drink, take a drug, or watch television).	4	3	2	1	0

(continued)

	How much do you believe it?				
	4 Totally	3 Very much	2 Mod-erately	1 Slightly	0 Not at all
8. I should avoid situations in which I attract attention, or be as inconspicuous as possible.	4	3	2	1	0
9. Unpleasant feelings will escalate and get out of control.	4	3	2	1	0
10. If others criticize me, they must be right.	4	3	2	1	0
11. It is better not to do anything than to try something that might fail.	4	3	2	1	0
12. If I don't think about a problem, I don't have to do anything about it.	4	3	2	1	0
13. Any signs of tension in a relationship indicate the relationship has gone bad; therefore, I should cut it off.	4	3	2	1	0
14. If I ignore a problem, it will go away.	4	3	2	1	0
15. I am needy and weak.	4	3	2	1	0
16. I need somebody around available at all times to help me to carry out what I need to do or in case something bad happens.	4	3	2	1	0
17. My helper can be nurturant, supportive, and confident—if he or she wants to be.	4	3	2	1	0
18. I am helpless when I'm left on my own.	4	3	2	1	0
19. I am basically alone—unless I can attach myself to a stronger person.	4	3	2	1	0
20. The worst possible thing would be to be abandoned.	4	3	2	1	0
21. If I am not loved, I will always be unhappy.	4	3	2	1	0
22. I must do nothing to offend my supporter or helper.	4	3	2	1	0
23. I must be subservient in order to maintain his or her goodwill.	4	3	2	1	0
24. I must maintain access to him or her at all times.	4	3	2	1	0
25. I should cultivate as intimate a relationship as possible.	4	3	2	1	0
26. I can't make decisions on my own.	4	3	2	1	0
27. I can't cope as other people can.	4	3	2	1	0
28. I need others to help me make decisions or tell me what to do.	4	3	2	1	0
29. I am self-sufficient, but I do need others to help me reach my goals.	4	3	2	1	0
30. The only way I can preserve my self-respect is by asserting myself indirectly (for example, by not carrying out instructions exactly).	4	3	2	1	0
31. I like to be attached to people but I am unwilling to pay the price of being dominated.	4	3	2	1	0
32. Authority figures tend to be intrusive, demanding, interfering, and controlling.	4	3	2	1	0

(continued)

	How much do you believe it?				
	4 Totally	3 Very much	2 Mod- erately	1 Slightly	0 Not at all
33. I have to resist the domination of authorities but at the same time maintain their approval and acceptance.	4	3	2	1	0
34. Being controlled or dominated by others is intolerable.	4	3	2	1	0
35. I have to do things my own way.	4	3	2	1	0
36. Making deadlines, complying with demands, and conforming are direct blows to my pride and self-sufficiency.	4	3	2	1	0
37. If I follow the rules the way people expect, it will inhibit my freedom of action.	4	3	2	1	0
38. It is best not to express my anger directly but to show my displeasure by not conforming.	4	3	2	1	0
39. I know what's best for me and other people shouldn't tell me what to do.	4	3	2	1	0
40. Rules are arbitrary and stifle me.	4	3	2	1	0
41. Other people are often too demanding.	4	3	2	1	0
42. If I regard people as too bossy, I have a right to disregard their demands.	4	3	2	1	0
43. I am fully responsible for myself and others.	4	3	2	1	0
44. I have to depend on myself to see that things get done.	4	3	2	1	0
45. Others tend to be too casual, often irresponsible, self-indulgent, or incompetent.	4	3	2	1	0
46. It is important to do a perfect job on everything.	4	3	2	1	0
47. I need order, systems, and rules in order to get the job done properly.	4	3	2	1	0
48. If I don't have systems, everything will fall apart.	4	3	2	1	0
49. Any flaw or defect of performance may lead to a catastrophe.	4	3	2	1	0
50. It is necessary to stick to the highest standards at all times, or things will fall apart.	4	3	2	1	0
51. I need to be in complete control of my emotions.	4	3	2	1	0
52. People should do things my way.	4	3	2	1	0
53. If I don't perform at the highest level, I will fail.	4	3	2	1	0
54. Flaws, defects, or mistakes are intolerable.	4	3	2	1	0
55. Details are extremely important.	4	3	2	1	0
56. My way of doing things is generally the best way.	4	3	2	1	0
57. I have to look out for myself.	4	3	2	1	0
58. Force or cunning is the best way to get things done.	4	3	2	1	0
59. We live in a jungle and the strong person is the one who survives.	4	3	2	1	0

(continued)

	How much do you believe it?				
	4 Totally	3 Very much	2 Mod- erately	1 Slightly	0 Not at all
60. People will get at me if I don't get them first.	4	3	2	1	0
61. It is not important to keep promises or honor debts.	4	3	2	1	0
62. Lying and cheating are okay as long as you don't get caught.	4	3	2	1	0
63. I have been unfairly treated and am entitled to get my fair share by whatever means I can.	4	3	2	1	0
64. Other people are weak and deserve to be taken.	4	3	2	1	0
65. If I don't push other people, I will get pushed around.	4	3	2	1	0
66. I should do whatever I can get away with.	4	3	2	1	0
67. What others think of me doesn't really matter.	4	3	2	1	0
68. If I want something, I should do whatever is necessary to get it.	4	3	2	1	0
69. I can get away with things so I don't need to worry about bad consequences.	4	3	2	1	0
70. If people can't take care of themselves, that's their problem.	4	3	2	1	0
71. I am a very special person.	4	3	2	1	0
72. Since I am so superior, I am entitled to special treatment and privileges.	4	3	2	1	0
73. I don't have to be bound by the rules that apply to other people.	4	3	2	1	0
74. It is very important to get recognition, praise, and admiration.	4	3	2	1	0
75. If others don't respect my status, they should be punished.	4	3	2	1	0
76. Other people should satisfy my needs.	4	3	2	1	0
77. Other people should recognize how special I am.	4	3	2	1	0
78. It's intolerable if I'm not accorded my due respect or don't get what I'm entitled to.	4	3	2	1	0
79. Other people don't deserve the admiration or riches they get.	4	3	2	1	0
80. People have no right to criticize me.	4	3	2	1	0
81. No one's needs should interfere with my own.	4	3	2	1	0
82. Since I am so talented, people should go out of their way to promote my career.	4	3	2	1	0
83. Only people as brilliant as I am understand me.	4	3	2	1	0
84. I have every reason to expect grand things.	4	3	2	1	0
85. I am an interesting, exciting person.	4	3	2	1	0
86. In order to be happy, I need other people to pay attention to me.	4	3	2	1	0
87. Unless I entertain or impress people, I am nothing.	4	3	2	1	0

(continued)

	How much do you believe it?				
	4 Totally	3 Very much	2 Mod- erately	1 Slightly	0 Not at all
88. If I don't keep others engaged with me, they won't like me.	4	3	2	1	0
89. The way to get what I want is to dazzle or amuse people.	4	3	2	1	0
90. If people don't respond very positively to me, they are rotten.	4	3	2	1	0
91. It is awful if people ignore me.	4	3	2	1	0
92. I should be the center of attention.	4	3	2	1	0
93. I don't have to bother to think things through—I can go by my "gut" feeling.	4	3	2	1	0
94. If I entertain people, they will not notice my weaknesses.	4	3	2	1	0
95. I cannot tolerate boredom.	4	3	2	1	0
96. If I feel like doing something, I should go ahead and do it.	4	3	2	1	0
97. People will pay attention only if I act in extreme ways.	4	3	2	1	0
98. Feelings and intuition are much more important than rational thinking and planning.	4	3	2	1	0
99. It doesn't matter what other people think of me.	4	3	2	1	0
100. It is important for me to be free and independent of others.	4	3	2	1	0
101. I enjoy doing things more by myself than with other people.	4	3	2	1	0
102. In many situations, I am better off to be left alone.	4	3	2	1	0
103. I am not influenced by others in what I decide to do.	4	3	2	1	0
104. Intimate relations with other people are not important to me.	4	3	2	1	0
105. I set my own standards and goals for myself.	4	3	2	1	0
106. My privacy is much more important to me than closeness to people.	4	3	2	1	0
107. What other people think doesn't matter to me.	4	3	2	1	0
108. I can manage things on my own without anybody's help.	4	3	2	1	0
109. It's better to be alone than to feel "stuck" with other people.	4	3	2	1	0
110. I shouldn't confide in others.	4	3	2	1	0
111. I can use other people for my own purposes as long as I don't get involved.	4	3	2	1	0
112. Relationships are messy and interfere with freedom.	4	3	2	1	0
113. I cannot trust other people.	4	3	2	1	0

(continued)

	How much do you believe it?				
	4 Totally	3 Very much	2 Moderately	1 Slightly	0 Not at all
114. Other people have hidden motives.	4	3	2	1	0
115. Others will try to use me or manipulate me if I don't watch out.	4	3	2	1	0
116. I have to be on guard at all times.	4	3	2	1	0
117. It isn't safe to confide in other people.	4	3	2	1	0
118. If people act friendly, they may be trying to use or exploit me.	4	3	2	1	0
119. People will take advantage of me if I give them the chance.	4	3	2	1	0
120. For the most part, other people are unfriendly.	4	3	2	1	0
121. Other people will deliberately try to demean me.	4	3	2	1	0
122. Oftentimes people deliberately want to annoy me.	4	3	2	1	0
123. I will be in serious trouble if I let other people think they can get away with mistreating me.	4	3	2	1	0
124. If other people find out things about me, they will use them against me.	4	3	2	1	0
125. People often say one thing and mean something else.	4	3	2	1	0
126. A person whom I am close to could be disloyal or unfaithful.	4	3	2	1	0

References

American Psychiatric Association. (1987). *Diagnostic and statistical manual of mental disorders* (3rd ed. rev.). Washington, DC: Author.

American Psychiatric Association. (2000). *Diagnostic and statistical manual of mental disorders* (4th ed. text rev.). Washington, DC: Author.

Asaad, G. (1995). *Understanding mental disorders due to medical conditions or substance abuse: What every therapist should know*. New York: Brunner/Mazel.

Beck, A. T. (1976). *Cognitive therapy and the emotional disorders*. New York: International Universities Press.

Beck, A. T. (2003). Synopsis of the cognitive model of borderline personality disorder. *Cognitive Therapy Today, 8*(2), 1–2.

Beck, A. T., & Beck, J. S. (1995). *The Personality Belief Questionnaire*. Bala Cynwyd, PA: Beck Institute for Cognitive Therapy and Research.

Beck, A. T., Butler, A. C., Brown, G. K., Dahlsgaard, K. K., Newman, C. F., & Beck, J. S. (2001). Dysfunctional beliefs discriminated personality disorders. *Behaviour Research and Therapy, 39*(10), 1213–1225.

Beck, A. T., Emery, G., & Greenberg, R. (1985). *Anxiety disorders and phobias: A cognitive perspective*. New York: Basic Books.

Beck, A. T., Epstein, N., Brown, G., & Steer, R. A. (1988). An inventory for measuring clinical anxiety: Psychometric properties. *Journal of Consulting and Clinical Psychology, 56*(6), 893-897.

Beck, A. T., Freeman, A., Davis, D. D., & Associates. (2004). *Cognitive therapy of personality disorders* (2nd ed.). New York: Guilford Press.

Beck, A. T., Rush, A. J., Shaw, B. F., & Emery, G. (1979). *Cognitive therapy of depression*. New York: Guilford Press.

Beck, A. T., Ward, C. H., Mendelson, M., Mock, J., & Erbaugh, J. (1961). An inventory for measuring depression. *Archives of General Psychiatry, 4*, 561–571.

Beck, A. T., Weissman, A., Lester, D., & Trexler, L. (1974). The measurement of pessimism: The Hopelessness Scale. *Journal of Consulting and Clinical Psychology, 42*(6), 861-865.

Beck, J. S. (1995). *Cognitive therapy: Basics and beyond.* New York: Guilford Press.

Beck, J. S. (1997). Personality disorders: Cognitive approaches. In L. J. Dickstein, M. B. Riba, & J. M. Oldham (Eds.), *American Psychiatric Press Review of Psychiatry, 16,* (pp. 73–106). Washington DC: American Psychiatric Press.

Beck, J. S. (2001). Reviewing therapy notes. In H. G. Rosenthal (Ed.), *Favorite counseling and therapy homework assignments* (pp. 37–39). Philadelphia, PA: Brunner-Routledge.

Beck, J. S. (2005). *Cognitive therapy worksheet packet (revised).* Bala Cynwyd, PA: Beck Institute for Cognitive Therapy and Research.

Beck, J. S., Beck, A. T., & Jolly, J. (2001). *Manual for the Beck Youth Inventories of Emotional and Social Impairment.* San Antonio, TX: The Psychological Corporation.

Butler, G., Cullington, A., Hibbert, G., Klimes, I., & Gelder, M. (1987). Anxiety management for persistent generalized anxiety. *British Journal of Psychiatry, 151,* 535–542.

Clark, D. A. (2004). *Cognitive-behavioral therapy for obsessive–compulsive disorder.* New York: Guilford Press.

Clark, D. A., Beck, A. T., & Alford, B. A. (1999). *Scientific foundations of cognitive theory and therapy of depression.* New York: Guilford Press

Clark, D. M., & Ehlers, A. (1993). An overview of the cognitive theory and treatment of panic disorder. *Applied and Preventive Psychology, 2*(3), 131–139.

Clark, D. M., & Wells, A. (1995). A cognitive model of social phobia. In R. G. Heimberg, M. Liebowitz, D. A. Hope, & F. A. Schneier (Eds.), *Social phobia: Diagnosis, assessment, and treatment* (pp. 69–93). New York: Guilford Press.

DeRubeis, R. J., & Feeley, M. (1990). Determinants of change in cognitive therapy for depression. *Cognitive Therapy and Research, 14,* 469–482.

Edwards, D. (1990). Cognitive therapy and the restructuring of early memories through guided imagery. *Journal of Cognitive Psychotherapy, 4*(1), 33–50.

Ellis, T. A., & Newman, C. F. (1996). *Choosing to live: How to defeat suicide through cognitive therapy.* Oakland, CA: New Harbinger Publications.

Franklin, M. E., & Foa, E. B. (2002). Cognitive behavioral treatments for obsessive compulsive disorder. In P. E. Nathan & J. M. Gorman (Eds.), *A guide to treatments that work* (2nd ed., pp. 367–386). London: Oxford University Press.

Freeman, A., & Reinecke, M. (1993). *Cognitive therapy of suicidal behavior: A manual for treatment.* New York: Springer.

Frost, R. O., & Skeketee, G. (Eds.). (2002). *Cognitive approaches to obsessions and compulsions: Theory, assessment, and treatment.* Elmont, NY: Pergamon Press.

Greenberger, D. G., & Padesky, C. A. (1995). *Mind over mood.* New York: Guilford Press.

Holmes, E. A., & Hackmann, A. (2004). *Mental imagery and memory in psychopathology.* Oxford, UK: Psychology Press.

Hopko, D. R., LeJuez, C. W., Ruggiero, K. J., & Eifert, G. H. (2003). Contemporary behavioral activation treatments for depression: Procedures, principles, and progress. *Clinical Psychology Review, 23*(5), 699–717.

Layden, M. A., Newman, C. F., Freeman, A., & Morse, S. B. (1993). *Cognitive therapy of borderline personality disorder.* Boston: Allyn & Bacon.

Leahy, R. L. (1996). *Cognitive therapy: Basic principles and applications.* Northvale, NJ: Aronson.

Leahy, R. L. (2001). *Overcoming resistance in cognitive therapy*. New York: Guilford Press.

Mahoney, M. (1991). *Human change processes*. New York: Basic Books.

McCullough, J. (2000). *Treatment for chronic depression: Cognitive behavioral analysis system of psychotherapy*. New York: Guilford Press.

McGinn, L. K., & Sanderson, W. C. (1999). *Treatment of obsessive-compulsive disorder*. Northvale, NJ: Jason Aronson.

McKay, M., & Fanning, P. (1991). *Prisoners of belief*. Oakland: New Harbinger Publications.

Meichenbaum, D., & Turk, D. C. (1987). *Facilitating treatment adherence*. New York: Plenum Press.

Millon, T., & Davis, R. D. (1996). *Disorders of personality: DSM-IV and beyond* (2nd ed.). New York: Wiley.

Moore, R., & Garland, A. (2003). *Cognitive therapy for chronic and persistent depression*. New York: Wiley.

Newman, C. F. (1991). Cognitive therapy and the facilitation of affect: Two case illustrations. *Journal of Cognitive Psychotherapy: An International Quarterly, 5*(4), 305–316.

Newman, C. F. (1994). Understanding client resistance: Methods for enhancing motivation to change. *Cognitive and Behavioral Practice, 1*, 47–69.

Newman, C. F. (1997). Maintaining professionalism in the face of emotional abuse from clients. *Cognitive and Behavioral Practice, 4*(1), 1–29.

Newman, C. F. (1998). The therapeutic relationship and alliance in short-term cognitive therapy. In J. Safran & J. C. Muran (Eds.), *The therapeutic alliance in brief psychotherapy* (pp. 95–122). Washington, DC: American Psychological Association.

Newman, C. F., & Ratto, C. (2003). Narcissistic personality disorder. In M. Reinecke & D. A. Clark (Eds.), *Cognitive therapy across the lifespan* (pp. 172–201). Cambridge, UK: Cambridge University Press.

Newman, C. F., & Strauss, J. L. (2003). When clients are untruthful: Implications for the therapeutic alliance, case conceptualization, and intervention. *Journal of Cognitive Psychotherapy: An International Quarterly, 17*(3), 241–252.

Padesky, C. A. (1993). Schema as self-prejudice. *International Cognitive Therapy Newsletter, 5/6*, 16–17.

Persons, J. B., Burns, B. D., & Perloff, J. M. (1988). Predictors of drop-out and outcome in cognitive therapy for depression in a private practice setting. *Cognitive Therapy and Research, 12*, 557–575.

Pope, K. S., Sonne, J. L., & Horoyd, J. (1993). *Sexual feelings in psychotherapy: Explorations for therapists and therapists-in-training*. Washington, DC: American Psychological Association.

Pretzer, J. L., & Beck, A. T. (1996). A cognitive theory of personality disorders. In J. F. Clarkin & M. F. Lenzenweger (Eds.), *Major theories of personality disorder* (pp. 36–105). New York: Guilford Press.

Safran, J. D., & Muran, J. C. (2000). *Negotiating the therapeutic alliance: A relational treatment guide*. New York: Guilford Press.

Schmidt, N. B., Joiner, T. E., Jr., Young, J. E., & Telch, M. J. (1995). The Schema Questionnaire: Investigation of psychometric properties and the hierarchical structure of a measure of maladaptive schemata. *Cognitive Therapy and Research, 19*(3), 295–321.

Smucker, M. R., & Dancu, C. V. (1999). *Cognitive-behavioral treatment for adult survivors of childhood trauma.* Northvale, NJ: Aronson.

Spring, J. A. (1996). *After the affair: Healing the pain and rebuilding trust when a partner has been unfaithful.* New York: Harper Perennial.

Thompson, A. (1990). *Guide to ethical practice in psychotherapy.* Oxford, UK: Wiley.

Torgersen, S., Kringlen, E., & Cramer, V. (2001). The prevalence of personality disorders in a community sample. *Archives of General Psychiatry, 58,* 590–596.

Wells, A. (1997). *Cognitive therapy of anxiety disorders: A practical manual and conceptual guide.* Chichester, UK: Wiley.

Wells, A. (2000). *Emotional disorders and metacognition: Innovative cognitive therapy.* New York: Wiley.

Wright, J. H., & Basco, M. R. (2001). *Getting your life back: The complete guide to recovery from depression.* New York: Free Press

Yalom, I. D. (1980). *Existential psychotherapy.* New York: Basic Books.

Young, J. E. (1999). *Cognitive therapy for personality disorders: A schema-focused approach* (3rd ed.). Sarasota, FL: Professional Resource Exchange.

Young, J. E., & Beck, A. T. (1980). *Cognitive therapy scale: Rating manual.* Bala Cynwyd, PA: Beck Institute for Cognitive Therapy.

Young, J. E., Klosko, J. S., & Weishaar, M. E. (2003). *Schema therapy: A practitioner's guide.* New York: Guilford Press.

Index